Dr. Siegal's Natural Fiber Permanent Weight-Loss Diet

Dr. Siegal's Natural Fiber Permanent Weight-Loss Diet

Sanford Siegal D.O., M.D.

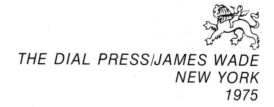

THE DIAL PRESS/JAMES WADE
NEW YORK
1975

Library of Congress Cataloging in Publication Data

Siegal, Sanford.
Dr. Siegal's natural fiber permanent
weight-loss diet.

Bibliography: p.
    1. High-fiber diet.   2. Reducing diets.
I. Title.
RM237.6.S53   613.2'5   75-28213
ISBN 0-8037-7803-1

Manufactured in the United States of America
First printing

ISBN 0-8037-7803-1

To Lyndol,
who knew I could

I want to express my gratitude to

Dan Abelow, for his totally dedicated editing and
preparation of the manuscript

Arlene Maranz, for her flawless typing

Juliette Beer, for her enthusiastic assistance with the
recipes

Ray Thorburn, a researcher *par excellence*

Clara Martin, Mercy Marrero, and Elaine Wood, for their
faithful assistance

Barry Feuerman, M.D., William Bronkan, D.D.S.,
Harold Unger, M.D., Lloyd Meisels, D.V.M.,
and Bernard Goldfarb, L.L.B. for their thoughtful
responses to my questions

Beth Anne Touchton, for her general supervision and
expertise with the calculator

And above all my wife, who tolerated turning our home
into a laboratory

To all of them, a very sincere Thank You

TO THE READER —
AND THE DIETER

Preventive medicine is the best medicine, but preventive medicine can't be accomplished unless you see your doctor on a regular basis. Although this is a perfectly natural diet based on good nutritional principles, and one I am recommending to my patients, I am not your doctor and I am not undertaking to treat you. This is your family doctor's province.

Before starting any diet you should consult your doctor and discuss the diet you intend to follow. He or she may have some good reasons why you should not diet or go on *this* diet. Also, he or she may be unaware of the new medical and scientific literature and research reports that form the very solid foundation of this diet. Accordingly, I would be delighted to furnish additional specific information to any fellow physician who would like to see it. My address is given in Chapter 9.

Sanford Siegal, D.O., M.D.

CONTENTS

CHAPTER 1

FACE IT, IT'S WAR

First of all, it's not your fault. You're not the villain, you're the innocent victim.

There is a medical breakthrough so new that most doctors haven't even heard about it. If you take advantage of it, by entirely natural means you will comfortably restore your weight to normal, leaving yourself as trim and healthy as you've always wanted to be. The information contained in this book is too important for you not to know, and you can begin using it *today*.

I will show you that it is not the food you are eating that has made you fat, but rather what you have not been eating. What you need to make you thin has not even been available to you.

For years you've been battling this problem alone or with the help of well-meaning doctors. But the diets you've been on before are wrong. They assumed that you could lose weight by cutting food out of your diet. At best they always left you feeling hungry. At worst they distorted and interfered with the natural and healthy balances of your body. And they always eventually failed. The creators of previous diets were ignorant of this basic new information. But now that I have this new information, I will tell you how *you will lose weight by adding something to your diet.*

This idea that there is something wrong with us, either mentally or physically, that our bodies just naturally get fat, is ridiculous. The processed foods available to us are the key to the problem. When you think about it, isn't it obvious? There is nothing basically wrong with us. Your overweight problem is in the very nature of the foods that are given to you.

In fact, most Americans *are* on a diet and they don't know it. The diet they are on is "starving" their bodies even when it makes them feel "satisfied." The average American is an unknowing victim of a nutritional economy that is inflationary in more ways than one. It makes you fat and it keeps your wallet thin.

You don't need crash diets. You don't need starvation. You certainly don't need a pinched family food budget. You need to return to nutritional sanity.

Equally important is a second discovery, that this same missing food in our diet, if it were included, would not only prevent obesity—it should also protect us from a wide variety of dread and common diseases, including

   ·   coronary artery disease, which causes the most frequent type of heart attack
   ·   cancer of the colon, the number-two killer among cancers and the most common form of cancer
   ·   diverticulitis and diverticulosis, suffered by one out of three Americans over age forty-five
   ·   polyps of the colon, an affliction that strikes one out of every five adults
   ·   peptic ulcer, gallstones, diabetes, and many other diseases

These diseases and obesity, taken together, form what virtually constitutes an epidemic that is ravaging our country from coast to coast. In the past few decades more than ten million Americans have died from these diseases. According to the current actuarial predictions, millions more will die in the coming years.

I will not mince words. Both obesity and this epidemic of other diseases appear to be unnecessary. A whole body of new evidence implies that these problems are caused by a deficiency in our diets, a deficiency that you can correct. If you follow the recommendations presented here, it is likely that neither you nor your family need be plagued by obesity or by this epidemic. But you need to know what the epidemic is and why we are suffering from it in order to avoid it.

That's what this book is all about, explaining these new findings, telling you how to use them to control your weight, improve your appearance, and preserve your health. I am giving you the story behind this new discovery so you will understand why your new diet will make such a big difference.

As you might imagine, the implications of these new findings are so important that within a short time they could and should bring rapid change to the food industry and completely alter the posture of medical science about the cause and treatment of many diseases.

Apart from helping you control your weight, this book's aim is to prolong your life and perhaps to help improve the health of our whole society. While it offers you a weight-loss program, it is not just another diet book. It is a book that also offers you an easily usable program for helping preserve your health and the health of your loved ones. In other words, this book may prolong your life and improve your health even if you are not overweight.

Let's face it, the new evidence has brought forth the startling possibility that we're in the middle of an unnecessary health crisis. It is tragic to suggest that millions of past deaths were premature, and that those whose bodies are failing them now are suffering in vain. Families who have been hit by this epidemic have been or are being crushed by catastrophic health expenses. It is again tragic to say that the billions they are spending to try and stay alive could have remained in their bank accounts—and that the health-insurance premiums of all of us could be lower because we all might be much healthier.

How long will we continue to suffer these diseases? The program recommended in this book, based on the new evidence, is the first one formulated by a physician who dedicates himself exclusively to the treatment of obesity. If you follow this program, which is very easy to do, my experience shows that you will lose your excess weight and that you will gain permanent control over your weight problem.

What is this new discovery all about? It is about the important role of a substance called dietary fiber. When the fiber has been removed from the foods you eat, you consume mainly "naked calories"; and the new evidence indicates that this destroys your health. When the fiber is restored, it helps you lose weight and keep your proper weight easily. Including fiber in your meals helps prevent a variety of diseases and may save your life. Once you have seen the evidence for yourself, you will agree: this will undoubtedly affect the eating habits of millions of people.

I am trained in medicine, not in military strategy. Yet even I recognize the folly of a one-man war. I can't win a single battle or the whole war alone. Only you can win your own personal victory, and as more and more Americans win their battles, the enemy's onslaught will gradually be reversed, and victory will be won.

Naked calories are the enemy. They are the calories that remain after the fiber has been removed from your food. Naked calories are produced by the refining of sugar and flour, and the damage is done when you include these substances in your diet. (From infancy, when we eat baby foods loaded with sugar, we become a nation of sugar addicts.) Once eaten, sugar and processed foods operate invisibly, within the lightless recesses of your digestive tract, sabotaging its proper functioning. They entice you to kill yourself with sweet offerings. Then, when you are firmly entrenched in the enemy's camp, naked calories slowly and systematically strip you of your health.

Most likely you bought this book because of your weight problem. Dietary fiber will help you lose weight, and lose it reasonably quickly—with fewer hunger pangs than you've ever felt before while dieting.

But you say that your weight problem is special? That you've tried everything and nothing works? I've seen a lot of special cases. As the medical director of nine clinics limited to the treatment of overweight patients, in the last seventeen years I and the doctors who work with me have seen 50,000 special cases. In fact, at present we are treating thousands of patients who represent every shape, size, age, and color. Let me tell you how we approach obesity. It should help you feel more confident.

Seeing 50,000 patients gives you a familiarity with every aspect of the weight problem and the diet. You recognize that each patient is different. Each one must be treated individually; yet you also see similarities. You begin to classify the patients into groups. You see that within these groups common measures can be taken to solve the problem.

Perhaps the most common problem, and the one this book will help you solve, is how difficult it is for most of us to lose weight and then keep from gaining it back. You see, when nothing you do seems to work, it hasn't been your problem alone. We've struggled with it as well.

For years research and development in the field of weight reduction has been rather stagnant. There have been a number of well-wishing, dedicated workers who have done lots of experiments, written lots of scientific papers, but there hasn't been much progress. They haven't even made a real dent in the problem. Obesity has remained a major problem of Americans, no matter what approach or special diets medical science has tried.

As a matter of fact, it is daily growing worse. I've read all the books and frankly, they have little new to say. For years I treated patients with conventional good medicine and in many cases saw nice positive results. The reason I didn't write a book on dieting before is because there was nothing truly new that I could add to the subject.

Finally there has been a breakthrough. It has been a long

time coming, but its potentials are so dramatic that it almost seems worth the wait. It explains why our society as a whole has the incurable problem of excess fat. This breakthrough gives you a new way to remove your extra weight and keep it off—a better way than ever before. And it reveals an unsuspected, easy way to fight some of our most dreaded and common diseases, ailments that you will go to war against when you use the carefully developed program offered in this book.

It is almost certain that one or another element of this epidemic will attack you during your life if you do not change your diet. If you are young, or if you are middle-aged or older but still in good health, you are lucky. But a battle for survival looms in your future. Unless you take action today, there is a high probability that you will fall into the enemy's clutches— and lose your personal battle for good health, and maybe even your life.

I hope that you are planning to live a long and healthy life. If you are, I can show you how to tighten your fist and prevent the precious sands of health from slipping through your fingers.

I will shortly be telling you about the new findings that back up this dramatic potential for increased health. It is these new findings, along with the weight control and health protection recommendations, that are the real message of this book. They could cause a revolution in our society's eating habits and our treatment of disease.

If you are one of the many people who has tried other diets and none of them has worked, this new diet should work for you. If you are someone who has used other diets successfully, this one will work just as well, but offers you improved health at the same time.

Dietary fiber is concerned with much more than losing weight. It has the potential of ending the epidemic that rages in our country. It may even save your life.

This is the most excited I've been in seventeen years over developments in this field. My entire professional life has been devoted to helping patients with weight problems. No matter how many I've helped, more have needed help than I have been able to reach. Finally, with this breakthrough, we have a real chance to conquer our weight problems, and at the same time bring new health and vitality to all Americans.

CHAPTER 2

THE BREAKTHROUGH
THAT CAN END OBESITY

Why do we get fat? Why does obesity appear to be inevitable for the majority of us? Is it a basic defect in the human organism? Are all the books you've bought and all the diets you've tried simply that much wasted effort?

Dr. T. L. Cleave makes an excellent point in *The Saccharine Disease.** He points out that no birth defect is present in more than one half of one percent of the population. In fact, he lists club foot as the most common birth defect, and this is found in only 4.2 out of every 1,000 live births. The incidence of all other known birth defects is lower than this.

The exact incidence of obesity is hard to calculate, but estimates in the vicinity of 50 percent of the Western world are considered reasonable. These figures indicate that more than 100 million Americans are overweight. If obesity were to be considered a birth defect, its incidence is totally out of proportion to every other birth defect. Dr. Cleave's conclusion is that obesity is not an hereditary defect, but an acquired condition.

The search for the "why" of obesity takes us to the study of animals and, more importantly, to people living in societies other than our own. It appears that we can generalize in saying that wild animals are not overweight. Given adequate sources of food, they generally maintain a rather ideal weight.

---

*The word saccharine does not refer to the artificial sweetener, saccharin, which is spelled without an "e." Saccharine means relating to sugar.

In addition, there are whole groups of people who are not overweight. Some societies have no obesity problem whatsoever. If there is a basic defect, how is it that America has it, that many other modern societies have it, but that a few societies have escaped it?

Who are these fortunate people? Extensive studies made of Zulu tribes who live in the rural areas of Natal, in Africa, indicate that they have virtually no obesity. This is true for both men and women. Studies such as this cast a dark shadow on the theory that obesity is a widespread, nearly unavoidable problem.

The study of societies that display a higher incidence of a health problem, or in the case of the Zulus, that show the common *absence* of a problem, is one of the most valuable tools of the medical researcher. This answers the question of whether obesity is an acquired social and cultural problem or an hereditary problem that is untreatable except by the painful struggles of countless individuals. If it is truly the plight of a society rather than the individual, there are new and better ways to treat it.

The absence of obesity is observed equally in other "primitive" tribes in Africa, as well as on other continents and islands around the world. It would seem that not only animals but also men and women living in a rather primitive state do not suffer from obesity.

What do the Zulus eat? Are fattening foods even available to them?

Some astonishing facts were revealed by an analysis of the eating habits of the rural Zulus. Their diet consists of 90 percent carbohydrates. This is a revelation that will raise a lot of eyebrows in the Western world, because we have been taught the evils of a high-carbohydrate diet. Furthermore, many of these rural Zulus work as sugarcane cutters. They are permitted to eat unlimited amounts of raw sugarcane. Since their work is very hard, they consume great quantities of the sugarcane. The rest of their diet consists of corn and beans, both of which are carbohydrates. If carbohydrates are the culprit in Western society, they are certainly not fattening for the rural Zulus.

Medical researchers noted this inconsistency. Why doesn't a high-carbohydrate diet cause a weight problem for the rural Zulus? How does their high-carbohydrate diet keep them thin, while ours puts pounds on us? If this sounds confusing to you, imagine the perplexity of the medical researchers who first discovered it!

Fortunately for us, these researchers wanted an explanation and kept looking until they found it. It was no easy search, for the answers weren't discovered in the diets of these rural Zulus. They were healthy. The answer was found nearby, in the cities and towns of urbanized southern Africa.

You see, other Zulus do not live in rural areas. Some live in towns and have a completely different way of life.

How are they different? The diet of the Zulus living in urban areas resembles our American diet. What is the result? Zulu men who live in urban areas have approximately the *same* incidence of obesity as that of American men, and the Zulu women suffer an incidence of obesity over *twice* that of American women. This is an entirely different health picture than that of the rural Zulus.

With statistics such as these, we are immediately compelled to look at what the urban Zulu eats. Urban Zulus eat many of the refined and packaged foods that we consume. Dr. Cleave supplies us with a very useful analysis of the diet of the urban Zulu. He eats 16 percent refined sugar as compared to only 1 percent in the rural population. The rest of his carbohydrates come mainly from grains, but they are in the form of refined white bread, while his rural cousin eats carbohydrates in the form of corn and beans. The urban Zulu eats 85 pounds of refined sugar a year. The rural Zulu eats only 6 pounds. The average American consumes over 100 pounds a year.

This comparison produced something completely unexpected. The researchers discovered that the diets of the urban

Zulus are very high in carbohydrates, but *lower* than that of their rural countrymen. The urban Zulus ate only 81 percent carbohydrates, compared to 90 percent in rural areas. So we have a situation where those who eat *less* carbohydrates suffer a very *high* incidence of obesity, while those who eat *more* carbohydrates have almost *no* obesity.

From this, you might decide to begin eating a high-carbohydrate diet as a means of losing weight. Don't try it. It won't work. You're going to have to read a few paragraphs more to find out why it would only increase your weight.

Once the urban-rural comparison had been made, the key to the puzzle was soon found. The researchers discovered that the rural people ate different kinds of carbohydrates than the urban people. We've already mentioned the unrefined-carbohydrate diet of the rural people: corn, beans, sugarcane, etc. The urban Zulus who suffer obesity eat a diet very similar to our own.

The researchers began by studying two groups with the same racial and geographical origins. They learned that obesity is high in the urban group that ate a diet high in *refined* carbohydrates, but obesity was rare in the group whose diet was high in *unrefined* carbohydrates.

By itself, the discovery that a different diet will reduce obesity to a low level would not be enough to create great interest among medical researchers. A conclusive finding that we shouldn't eat refined carbohydrates might create a controversy because it would affect several big industries, but even that wouldn't create new excitement among scientists.

Yet this new excitement has started, and it is rapidly growing in momentum and breadth. In the following chapters I am going to tell you not to eat refined carbohydrates; but if it were only for the reason of keeping you from getting fat, I would have said it on the first page of the book. There are even more compelling reasons for not eating these foods.

If you think your only problem is that you're overweight,

you're wrong. The real breakthrough in the urban versus rural Zulus was that the urban people had disease rates very similar to the other urban people with whom they lived, but the rural Zulus were *much healthier.*

Just how much healthier is so astounding that a large part of the world of medical research is beginning to react seriously to it. If the evidence becomes generally known, it will produce a revolution in our eating habits.

I know you are reading these facts and are momentarily impressed with their implications, but because they concern Africans with whom your only contact may be through the pages of the *National Geographic,* you may try to dismiss them by saying that it is probably the result of some exotic characteristic of these distant people. However, this evidence does include us, as well as these "primitive" peoples. Before I spell out the whole story, a review of our own eating habits is quite revealing.

The latter half of the nineteenth century in the United States was marked by a shift from the use of crude brown sugar to the highly refined sugar that sits on our tables today. This was made possible by a new technology that enabled white sugar to be produced at a price not much higher than brown sugar. By the beginning of the twentieth century, there was, as happens in American industry, a virtual monopoly on the production of white sugar in this country. Furthermore, its widespread use was greatly stimulated by advertising, which showed enlarged photographs of insects supposedly present in brown sugar.

The extent to which our sugar consumption has changed turns out to be surprisingly large when we look at some actual figures. In the 1700s the sugar consumption in Great Britain was only 4 to 5 pounds a year per person. In the mid-1800s, this amount had multiplied to about 25 pounds a year per person. In 1970 this figure reached 120 pounds per person.

In our country, with the new inexpensive refined sugar, the consumption of sugar per individual doubled between 1880 and 1915. Today it is over 100 pounds per person each year. This quantity is so great that almost one out of every five calories that we eat each day comes from refined sugar.

At the same time that the refining of sugar began in the late 1800s, flour underwent a similar change. If you examine a grain of wheat you'll find that it contains three areas. Its outer coat is generally known as bran. The major part of the grain is the endosperm. This is the part that is ground into white flour. At the very center of the grain is the wheat germ, which contains a high percentage of oil as well as certain important vitamins. If the entire wheat grain is ground up, the resulting flour is beige in color. It is obtainable today as whole wheat flour.

During the end of the last century the flour processor's goal was to produce a pure white flour free of bran and free of the wheat germ, for the oil present in both these portions becomes rancid in time. They sought a new white flour that would store better and have a long shelf-life. Ingenuity and technology prevailed, and the old stone grinding mills were gradually replaced by new mills with metal rollers that very efficiently separated the "undesirable" portions of the wheat from the endosperm. The result was a pure white flour that could be made into pure white bread, light and fluffy in character, with a pleasant, sweet taste.

The use of flour did not increase in the late 1800s and the early 1900s; in fact, it dropped drastically. The whole wheat flour commonly eaten until the middle of the nineteenth century was discontinued and was only partially replaced by refined white flour.

Today our bread is made from refined white flour, which is the starchy endosperm remaining after the inner wheat germ and the outer bran coat have been removed. Of course, we all know that wheat germ is full of vitamins. To make up for the removal of the wheat germ, the federal government requires wheat processors to add vitamins to "enrich" their flour.

The bran coating of the wheat is also removed. This is not nearly as rich in vitamins as the wheat germ, but it is made up of the highest proportion of indigestible material. This indigestible material is generally referred to as fiber. It is also described as crude fiber or dietary fiber. Although some animals are able to derive nourishment from it, humans cannot.

Almost all of America's food research attempts to improve the quantity and quality of the nutrients food contains. No one cares about the indigestible fiber that has been removed from our food. We are concerned with getting high-quality carbohydrates and proteins. We make sure our fats are polyunsaturated rather than saturated, and we see to it that our diet contains sufficient vitamins and minerals.

The public and food researchers have become so engrossed in discussing the food additives, the preservatives, chemicals, insect specks, insecticides, proteins, and calories that are in our dinner that they have ignored one of the most important parts of food. Who would dream that the nonnutritive parts of our diet, the fiber, would prove more important that the nutritive portion? But that is exactly the case.

It is the nonnutritive portion of food that determines whether you are fat or thin. I shall explain why this is so, in detail, in Chapter 5. As I shall also show later, this fiber can determine whether you are healthy or sick, and even whether you live or die.

In the medical research on the Zulus, the breakthrough was the discovery that a number of diseases that are common both in our society and among urban Zulus are *almost nonexistent among rural Zulus.*

How can this be? Exactly what is this fiber that the rural Zulus eat?

All living things are made of many, many cells. A complicated animal like a human being contains literally billions of cells. Plants, such as vegetables and wheat, are also composed of huge numbers of cells.

A cell is like a container that is made of an outer shell and filled with a liquid or semi-liquid substance. In animals, the cell wall is very thin and flexible. In many plants, but not all of them, the cell's outer wall is stiff and hard. The material from which the plant cell wall is made is called cellulose.

When we eat plant foods, the stiff and hard cell walls are not actually a food, but rather the container that holds the food. The plant's carbohydrates, proteins, and fats are found within the more liquid portions of the cell. Yet this indigestible cell wall, the fiber, is the substance that is emerging as one of the most important parts of the food we eat.

Fiber is present in varying amounts in every plant that grows out of the ground. Wheat bran, for example contains very high amounts, as much as 12 percent, while tomatoes contain relatively small amounts, often less than 1 percent.

It is this fibrous cell wall that differentiates the food of the rural Zulus from that of the urban Zulus. The healthy, nonobese rural Zulu gets his fiber from the unrefined foods in his diet. He eats about 25 grams of fiber a day.

Americans and the urban Zulu eat mainly refined diets, one in which most of the fiber has been removed. In this country, we commonly eat 3 to 5 grams of fiber a day. As I will show, it is this fiber that makes the difference between a society without weight problems and an obese society.

I am also going to explain why the lack of fiber in your diet causes your personal weight problem, and why it is important that your weight-loss regime include the addition of fiber to your diet. If you attempt to follow any other means of losing weight, even though you may appear to be successful, you will not have gotten to the real cause of your excess weight. And if you don't add fiber to your diet, you will eventually return to your previous obese state. Most important, you will have done nothing to prevent a host of ailments that might make you ill before many years have passed, and could eventually kill you.

You will see that the evidence is unquestionable. Fiber will become the magic word in nutrition in the future, just as it has always been an essential element in digestion in the past.

The human digestive system did not evolve on the diet of refined carbohydrates that is common in our country today.

From our earliest four-foot tall, hairy, animal-skin-clad fore-bears through our great-great-grandparents, humanity's "grocery store" was the field and forest, not the modern super-market and the food-processing factories that stand behind it.

For millions of years every plant food eaten by humans was picked in the forest and field and either eaten directly or brought back to the cave, hut, or village. There it might have been pounded or cooked before it was eaten. Perhaps the wheat was winnowed in the wind, so the chaff would be blown away while the grain remained. But little more was done to food before it was eaten.

Until just a few decades ago every person consumed a diet high in fiber. There was no way to remove this fiber. If you wanted to eat, if you wanted to stay alive, you ate a great deal of plant foods, and your diet contained a high percentage of fiber.

The natural abundance of fiber forced a responsive evolution in the human digestive system. The normal human diet has always been high in fiber, and our digestive systems evolved to rely on this common part of food, even though it only passes through our bodies and emerges in a form quite similar to that which it entered. Today the human digestive system still requires sufficient amounts of fiber with each meal if it is to work properly and stay healthy.

As voluminous medical research points out, those peoples living in "primitive" surroundings and eating the unrefined diets of their ancestors do not suffer from a variety of diseases which have reached epidemic proportions in our "modern" so-ciety. Clearly, there is more than a message we should hear. There is a lesson we can learn.

It is a lesson to which we must pay attention if we are to regain the part-fiber, part-nutrient balance on which our diges-tive systems depend and rid ourselves of a major cause of those diseases which are needlessly killing millions and rob-bing all of us of billions of dollars in unnecessary health-care and insurance expenses.

In the next three chapters I will show you exactly why consuming dietary fiber should make you healthier, how its absence appears to cause disease, and how adding fiber to your diet should help prevent both obesity and a variety of diseases.

CHAPTER 3

THE CASE AGAINST OUR NUDE ADVERSARY – THE EPIDEMIC WE CAN STOP

Sam S. was referred to me six months ago by his family doctor for a program of weight reduction. He had been told that he had a disease he had never heard of before: diverticulitis. He suffered frequent, severe abdominal pains, and his doctor's treatments hadn't been working sufficiently well to clear up his condition. Fortunately, in the course of his weight-losing regime, his symptoms improved, but Sam is not cured. His weight problem was solved with a carefully designed program, but his large intestine has been permanently ruined by a lifetime of eating the wrong foods.

Diverticulosis and diverticulitis are two diseases you have probably never heard anything about. Yet one out of three Americans over the age of forty-five and two thirds of all Americans over eighty suffer from one or the other. They are serious diseases—and one remedy for acute cases is the surgical removal of the colon, an operation called a colostomy. The colon is the last intestinal tube through which food passes before it leaves the body. After a colostomy, what is left of the large intestine is attached to a hole cut into the patient's side. A bag is permanently attached to this hole. The odor, the discomfort, and the embarrassment that must be endured for the rest of the patient's life are an unavoidable result of this treatment.

What is the predominant cause of these two diseases? Evidence indicates that it is the diet we commonly eat.

The weight-loss diet offered in this book is based on this evidence, and the diet can do more than strip away your excess pounds—it can help protect you from succumbing to these diseases. This medical diet offers such dramatic health benefits that I hope it helps generate a public discussion that will convince the medical profession to act rapidly and save lives.

This is the second aim of this book: to provide greater health and well being for Americans who want it. Together we might save billions of dollars a year in unnecessary medical expenses. To make this goal a reality, there must be a specific change in the eating habits of our society, a dietary change that will be spelled out in coming chapters.

The medical professions have talked about the prevention of disease for a long, long time. If our nation could cut its hospital admissions by one fourth (which in my opinion my dietary program might accomplish), we would lift an enormous burden from the shoulders of the hospitals, insurance companies, and the public.

Our medical insurance premiums would be lowered. Doctors' offices would not be overcrowded, and our nation's shortage of doctors could be alleviated. We might find that we have enough doctors to provide better care for the diseases that remain. When insurance premiums are lowered, large employers who now pay huge insurance premiums might hold down the price of their products, helping slow our inflationary spiral.

Can all this really be accomplished by stopping one epidemic? The evidence that you are about to read says "Yes!" And it explains why our society needs to undergo a rapid dietary revolution.

The food we eat has already been through one revolution. Today it is very different from the unprocessed food eaten throughout all human prehistory and history, up until one hundred years ago. The defibered composition and chemical additives in today's food are even substantially changed from that eaten only forty or seventy years ago. Increasingly, over the last century, we have processed and refined our food more and more, to remove as much of the vegetable fiber as possible.

Our society's decision to refine its food was equivalent to leaping off the edge of a cliff into a seemingly bottomless pit, a pit of declining health. Fortunately, we remembered to strap on a parachute so that we would fall just slowly enough that scientists, doctors, and statisticians could document each new disease as it became prevalent, and devise treatments that would stave off, but not cure, the worst effects of these diseases.

Now, as we are falling slowly, new evidence from around the world has suddenly reached out and snagged our parachute on a branch protruding from the side of the pit. Our decision—whether or not we make this dietary change—will remove us entirely from this pit of declining health, or disentangle our parachute lines and force us to fall to the bottom.

Amazingly enough, the new evidence that snagged us may also give us the means to avoid a premature death and escape to a society of greatly improved weight control and better health.

How true is this illustration? Are we really halfway into a pit of declining health? Do we really have the chance to reverse our fall and return to full health?

Since facts and evidence show that the removal of fiber is causing major health problems in our society, let us look at the epidemiological evidence which supports these statements.

Two new questions are keeping medical researchers busy around the globe. What is the prevalence of disease among groups who include fiber in their diet, and how does their health compare with ours, now that we have removed the fiber? And we have substituted refined carbohydrates (sugar and white flour) for fibrous foods. Do these refined foods damage our health even more?

So you can easily have a total view of our declining health, I will tell you in advance where I'm heading. Then I will look at each of the diseases in turn and fit the evidence together into a complete picture.

A number of extremely serious diseases, as well as some very common ones, appear to have a common cause—the removal of fiber combined with the substitution of refined and processed foods. Medically, different ailments that have a single cause are thought of as one disease. Since the evidence shows this single, combined disease is frightfully widespread, I have called it an epidemic. And to give this epidemic a name, I have called it the Naked Calorie Disease.

From constipation to cancer, from ulcers to heart attacks, the Naked Calorie Disease robs us of tens of billions of dollars we cannot afford, money spent for the treatments we buy to cure its many subdiseases. It robs us of sound sleep at night as we toss and turn, trying to ignore the agonies of infected intestines or the fearful anxieties of living with cancer or heart disease.

Many of the ailments of the Naked Calorie Disease are *degenerative* diseases. As we begin to suffer them, our minds race to escape the emotional pressures of prematurely failing health. In its total impact, our lives are impoverished financially and emotionally by the Naked Calorie Disease, which often turns out to be our executioner.

The world's evidence points straight at our society's refining and processing of foods, and the cost is staggering.

Admittedly, these are drastic statements. They imply that our nation needs far more than a new system for losing weight. They suggest that our society needs to turn boldly to unprocessed foods in order to attempt to obtain the higher level of health and emotional well-being that almost everyone can enjoy.

VARICOSE VEINS

While varicose veins are perhaps not the most serious disease related to the removal of dietary fiber, they are a condition that can eventually affect every one of us. More than twenty million Americans already have varicose veins, and millions more will suffer from them during their lives.

These greatly enlarged blood vessels of the legs are a real potential danger to life. The blood is greatly slowed as it passes through these veins. Clots may then form which, when dislodged, move through the body and can cause strokes in the heart or lungs.

Because this condition is so common in America, some doctors assume that the same condition is equally common around the world. They believe that varicose veins are an unavoidable hereditary defect.

Others feel that varicose veins are an evolutionary defect produced when the human animal first stood erect. This opinion states that the blood vessels of the legs have never fully adapted to the standing position and these veins fail to provide adequate circulation.

When we step away from American doctors looking at American patients, extensive world evidence and a more logical view appears. This view asserts that it is the contents of the large intestine that actually create the problem.

Let us examine the evidence of a group of doctors, writing in *The British Medical Journal,* on a study of the transit time of food through the intestine. Transit time is the time it takes food to pass through your body. They reported that in a hospital in Zululand in Natal, South Africa, the transit times of patients there varied from twenty-four to forty-eight hours. More studies in Western countries indicate that the transit time of food through the intestinal tract is forty-eight to ninety-six hours.

Dr. Denis Burkitt, of The British Medical Research Council, reported in the esteemed medical journal *Lancet* on a large study of 1,000 subjects of varying ethnic groups. These included British boarding-school children, rural African villagers, and British vegetarians. He showed that the more refined the diet, the smaller the stool and the slower the passage of food through the intestine.

It was also noted that the longer transit times from refined foods could be shortened. When the Western subjects were fed high-fiber diets, the transit time decreased.

Our normal, low-fiber, refined-foods diet produces a prolonged transit time of the stool through our intestinal tract. By the time the stool reaches the end portions of the large intestine—the descending colon—it is quite dehydrated, well formed, and hard. In the upright position this hard stool exerts considerable pressure against the veins of the lower extremeties. Because of its slow transit speed, the stool often remains in the lower intestine for a long time and exerts pressure on these veins for a prolonged period. This pressure causes slowing of the blood in the veins, and this expands them. Over the years this weakens and finally destroys the valves and walls in the veins of the left leg.

When we study the African who lives in a more "primitive" society, we discover that his high-fiber diet results in a much shorter transit time for food through his intestinal tract. In fact, it takes an African half the time to get rid of his food than it does people in our country. The African's stools are larger, weighing twice as much. But they are soft and generally unformed. The result is that there is less pressure against his veins, and this pressure is exerted for a shorter period of time.

The key to proving every scientific theory is how well it predicts what happens in the real world. If our theory is correct, we would expect that Africans, who eat a high-fiber diet, to have a smaller incidence of varicose veins than we have in America.

Not only is this the case, but the differences between their societies and ours is dramatic. Over a three-year period 11,462 patients were admitted to a hospital in the Zululand Reserve in South Africa. In addition, the hospital treated 103,857 patients on an outpatient basis. Of all these patients, there were only *three* reported cases of varicose veins. In a similar group in the United States we would expect to see well over 10,000 cases.

Some may look at these statistics and say that since we are dealing with different races, other factors may explain the differences. They may say that we are comparing the black population of Africa with a predominantly white population in the

United States. But the incidence of varicose veins among the black population of the United States is virtually the same as that among white Americans. The ancestors of all American blacks came to this country from Africa less than three hundred and fifty years ago. Three centuries is not sufficient time to explain evolutionary changes. And for those who might argue that the African blacks do much harder physical labor than those in America, we can only reply that there is a rather large number of black Americans who are compelled to do hard physical labor.

If you suspect the Zululand study mentioned above presents a unique phenomenon, let me assure you that it is not. For example, one worker studied 30,000 outpatients in another hospital in Africa. He found only one case of varicosities.

Dr. Burkitt relates how he personally examined 4,000 adults in Central Africa and detected only five cases of varicose veins. This was only 1 percent of the number that he would have detected in a like group in Great Britain.

A medical questionnaire was sent to doctors in 114 hospitals in Africa. Seventy-eight percent of the doctors estimated that they saw less than five patients a year with varicose veins.

Questionnaires sent to hospitals in India and Pakistan, in areas where high-fiber diets are also eaten, indicated a similar low incidence of varicose veins.

A common complication of varicosities are ulcers that develop in the legs. These are routinely treated in hospitals throughout our country. A study of 9,000 patients in Iran who exist mainly on a diet of unrefined wheat and barley yielded not a single case of leg ulcer.

The application of this information to prevent varicose veins in our country is very slow in coming. Despite overwhelming evidence, there seems to be a general apathy when it comes to implementing the obvious.

In his book, Dr. Cleave reports on a previously uncommon use of dietary fiber by a hospital in England. A frequent complication after surgery is the formation of blood clots in the legs.

Various techniques have been devised to keep this from occurring, because these blood clots can cause fatal strokes. Dr. Cleave reports that in a particular ward in a hospital in England post-operative patients were put on a high-fiber diet where the fiber was supplied by bran. In over eighteen months there wasn't a single case of blood clots in the leg.

If you are impressed by the revelation that an ailment affecting 10 percent of our population can be eradicted in a relatively simple way, try to contain your enthusiasm. I have barely scratched the surface.

DIVERTICULAR DISEASE

I would wager that most people have not heard of diverticular disease. Yet it is one of the most common diseases affecting the American people. Why the popular magazines have chosen to ignore it, when it affects one out of every three people over age forty-five, is a mystery. I suppose there is nothing romantic about a disease of the large intestine, and therefore it doesn't make good reading. Nonetheless, if you are over forty-five, or if you hope to be healthy when you are older than forty-five, there is one chance in three that diverticulitis will strike you, unless . . .

Actually, I am talking about a lifelong chain of cause and effect, the more severe disease growing out of the less severe, the less severe growing out of our eating habits. The parent disease is diverticulosis, and diverticulitis develops from it. The colon, which is the muscular tube that carries your food in its final hours in your body, is the site of this problem. There are many theories as to the origin of the disease. Because of substantial epidemiological evidence, I accept the following.

The average American eats processed food during his entire lifetime. His stools are hard, dry, slow-moving dehydrated lumps. He believes this is normal because everyone eats this way, and because he expects his bowel movements to come like clockwork, and they often do. But he also has to resort to laxatives occasionally—sometimes often. In fact, laxatives are a $300 million a year business in our country.

In order for the large intestine to move these hard stools, the muscles in the walls of the colon must exert tremendous pressure. On a day-to-day basis, the effects of these exertions on the colon are not obvious. Diverticulosis is not a disease that develops in one day. Indeed, the incubation period is generally at least thirty years, and in most people it is over forty years. So after forty years of this tremendous strain on the colon, the muscle fibers begin to separate. Then the soft lining of the colon begins to form pockets that rupture through the muscular walls of the intestine. The end result is the formation of diverticuli, which are "blind pouches" that protrude from the wall of the intestines.

These pouches trap fecal material and bacteria within them. They harbor pieces of stool that support bacterial growth for lengthy periods. When this happens, the pouch becomes infected. This condition is known as diverticulitis, the medical term for inflammation of the diverticuli.

The symptoms are abdominal pain and soreness, sometimes quite severe, and the physician who is consulted often confuses this ailment for appendicitis, although in the majority of cases the symptoms are present on the left side, whereas appendicitis usually shows its pain on the right side.

Indeed, patients are often taken to surgery only to discover after the abdominal wall has been cut and the patient will bear a scar for the rest of his life that the condition was diverticulitis and not appendicitis.

Actually, appendicitis and diverticulitis are rather similar. Both may result from food becoming trapped in a blind pouch. The difference is that the appendix is normal and present at birth—and if it becomes infected, it can be removed without further complications. The diverticuli, the "little appendices," take forty years of persistent bad eating habits to develop, but once they have formed, there is no way to remove them. There is always the colostomy as a last resort, but living with a bag attached to a hole in your side, into which your stool involuntarily pours, is a dubious cure. The only hope is a treatment designed to hold down the symptoms, but there is no certainty that this treatment will work.

For years the diet prescribed for diverticulosis and diverticulitis was the low-residue diet. The aim was to have present as little residual material as possible to become trapped in the blind pouches. Recently, the absolute opposite treatment has been put into practice. Increasingly, large numbers of doctors are realizing that the treatment of choice is the *high* residue diet, particularly as a preventive treatment. The object of this new treatment is to get the food through the intestinal tract as quickly as possible. The shorter the time that it remains within the intestine the softer the stool, the less strain there is on the colon, and the less bacterial growth that occurs. In fact, the high-fiber diet recommended in this book is the ideal one for the prevention of diverticulitis.

A study was made of 200 hospitals in twenty countries. It revealed that diverticular disease, appendicitis, and malignant tumors in the colon are rare in the developing countries where foods are unrefined. It also showed that when refined foods are introduced into a developing country, the incidence of these diseases increased; but in the case of diverticular disease, there is often a very long period of time before the increase shows up. This is because of the thirty- to forty-year incubation period for the disease.

Dr. Burkitt, in association with Dr. Neil Painter, reported in another article in *The British Medical Journal* that the incidence of diverticular disease has increased dramatically in the last seventy years. Since it is so recent, it can hardly be dubbed a genetic defect.

At the turn of the century, diverticular disease was virtually unknown. Indeed, many medical textbooks of that time made no mention of it. Today, it affects one third of the Western population over age forty-five. By the time we reach the age of eighty, two thirds of us have it. The fact that it began to make its appearance around 1900 is very suspicious, since the whole-sale refining of flour began about thirty years before that date.

Dr. Burkitt stated that he performed surgery routinely over a period of twenty years in African hospitals and never saw a single case of diverticular disease.

A hospital in Kampala, Uganda, reported only two cases of diverticular disease in 4,000 autopsies. More reports come from parts of Asia where the condition is equally rare.

I would venture to say that any intern in an American hospital, fresh out of school, on his or her first day in surgical service, will see cases of diverticular disease.

The evidence is overwhelming that diverticular disease is caused by a lack of fiber in our diets. In the Western world it is present in both blacks and whites—and in about the same proportion. Among the African blacks who do not eat processed foods, and in developing countries where people eat high-fiber diets, there is no significant incidence of diverticular disease.

Since this is another widespread ailment that, like varicose veins, can be prevented by a fairly simple dietary change, your enthusiasm is probably growing by leaps and bounds. But hold yourself together for a little longer. The big guns are now ready to start firing.

CORONARY ARTERY DISEASE

Of all kinds of heart disease, coronary artery disease is the leading cause of heart attacks.

Heart disease is the greatest single cause of premature death in most Western nations. It takes more lives than respiratory illnesses, cerebrovascular disease, and all accidents. We all fear cancer, but in America, heart disease takes twice as many lives.

Many researchers have found a direct link between heart disease and the industrialization of a nation. When developing countries industrialize, the rate of heart disease goes up sharply. The blame is usually put on a rising consumption of animal fat.

In fact, there has been so much emphasis put on the role of animal fat and cholesterol as the cause of heart disease that most researchers have not looked in other directions. This dedication to cholesterol may be killing many Americans, because there are major inconsistencies that tend to contradict this theory. For example, Eskimos eat tremendous amounts of animal fat in the form of blubber and whale oil—but they have a very low incidence of heart disease.

A second major contradiction is that there has been a sudden acceleration in the number of deaths from coronary disease in this country, yet there has been no great increase in the consumption of animal fats. There has been a marked increase in the consumption of fats, but a major part of these fats have been the unsaturated vegetable ones, which are supposed to protect against coronary disease. Even though the consumption of animal fat has not risen enormously and the use of vegetable fats has increased, the crude death rate from heart disease rose from 79 per million persons in 1930 to 2,900 per million in 1963.

During this period the amount of fiber eaten fell enormously, and the amount of sugar consumed rose. But I will come back to these factors in a moment.

Just what is coronary artery disease? The heart is a muscular organ that not only pumps blood to the entire body, but pumps blood to itself for its own nourishment. Without this nourishment, the heart dies, and death of the whole body follows rapidly.

The heart feeds itself through two blood vessels called coronary arteries. The most common form of heart attack occurs when one or both of the coronary arteries becomes either partially or completely blocked. This blockage is caused by cholesterol and lipids depositing themselves on the inside walls of the two coronary arteries. As these fatty deposits grow, they cause decreased blood flow to the heart.

When the blood flow to the heart is interrupted, the person generally feels a severe pain in the chest. It becomes hard to breathe, and any breathing that occurs comes only in short gasps. Inside the chest, the heart is malfunctioning, either by developing an abnormal rhythm, or in extreme cases, by not beating at all.

This kind of heart attack may cause permanent damage to the heart. It almost always kills some tissue in the area where the blood flow was stopped. This dead area is known as a myocardial infarction, a medical term you may have heard.

The medical names for this kind of heart disease are ischemic heart disease (ischemic refers to lack of blood flow), and atherosclerotic heart disease. In this book I will use the term coronary artery disease.

Around the world, the incidence of coronary artery disease parallels the occurrence of diverticular disease. For the most part, when discussing the distribution, you can substitute the words coronary artery disease for diverticular disease and there will only be a few inconsistencies. When there is a high incidence of diverticular disease, there is also a high incidence of coronary disease, and vice versa. This is strong evidence of a common cause.

Like diverticulitis, coronary artery disease appears to have a forty-year incubation period. The incidence of coronary artery disease seems to climb suddenly forty years after the fiber consumption of a population decreases.

But not everyone is ready to believe new implications, no matter how clear a picture they paint. For these people, I offer the following facts.

At the Pretoria Bantu Hospital, South Africa, there was one patient with coronary artery disease in 1969, three in 1970, and five in 1971. Compare this with our American hospitals, where a major function of the hospital is to treat coronary artery disease.

Near Johannesburg, South Africa, at the Baragwanath Hospital, over 40,000 Bantu native patients are admitted annually. During a recent eleven-year study of these admissions, there were only thirty patients with coronary artery disease, an average of less than three a year out of total hospital admissions of more than 440,000 patients.

Reports of 137 hospitals in twenty African countries where high-fiber diets are eaten predominantly indicated a similarly low incidence of coronary artery disease. Ninety-four doctors questioned stated that they had never diagnosed a case of coronary artery disease. Were they bad diagnosticians, or were they telling us that this disease is rare in societies that eat the foods that keep people healthy?

Interestingly enough, in the large towns and cities of southern Africa, where the black population eats a more Westernized diet, there is a surprisingly large number of cases of coronary artery disease. This is true, for instance, in Capetown and Johannesburg.

What about the symptoms that American doctors tell us precede heart attacks? Even among those people whom our doctors would call high-risk cases, a high-fiber diet apparently offers protection. A 1972 *British Medical Journal* article reported that coronary artery disease was seldom seen in Africans who were obese, had high blood pressure, and diabetes.

Your doctor uses these "preliminary signs" to inform you that your risk of heart attack is high. These signs also exist in a small percentage of the population in societies where a high-fiber diet is eaten. But they still exist. Yet when Dr. Denis Burkitt sent questionnaires to 36 hospitals in high-fiber eating areas of India and Pakistan, 16 out of the 36 hospitals reported they had never diagnosed a case of coronary thrombosis.

What about animal fats? A study done in India is revealing. An article in *The British Medical Journal* in 1967 reported on a group of railway workers in southern India who eat very little animal fat. Their diet is mainly polished rice, which contains very little fiber. Coronary artery disease is common among these railway workers. But in the other end of India, in the north, railway workers on a high-fiber diet of whole wheat, dhal, and beans—whose diet is high in animal fat—have very little coronary disease.

Feeding a high-fiber diet to rats has been shown to triple the cholesterol output of the stool over a no-residue diet. Interestingly enough, although the fiber was natural, unprocessed fiber, when purified cellulose was used, it had no effect.

The most reasonable explanation of this is that the high fiber intake increases the output of cholesterol in the stools. Regardless of what the person takes in, less of the cholesterol is absorbed and more leaves with the stool.

This has been proved first by analysis of the stool, and second, by the fact that a high-fiber diet does lower the blood cholesterol. Studies have been done that show that just the eating of bread, even if it isn't the highest fiber type of bread, lowers blood cholesterol.

This lowering of blood cholesterol levels through high fiber intake is an important finding. Perhaps equally important was the discovery that high-fiber diets reduce the formation of fatty deposits on the inside of the coronary arteries in laboratory animals. These fatty deposits are called atheroma plaques; they are made of cholesterol and lipids, and, by obstructing the arteries, they reduce the blood flow to the heart muscle. A high-fiber diet reduced the formation of these atheroma plaques even when the experimental animals were fed a high-fat diet.

The artificially high blood sugar levels resulting from the large amounts of processed carbohydrates in the Western diet may produce degenerative changes in the lining of the arteries, predisposing them to the cholesterol and fat deposits that eventually pave the way to thrombosis. High blood sugar is a warning sign of diabetes. The link between diabetes and coronary artery disease seems obvious. As Dr. Cleave emphatically affirms, "Of one thing the author is very confident; the key to causation of coronary thrombosis lies in the causation of diabetes (and also of obesity)."

I hope the point is beginning to come home to you. Animal fats and cholesterol may not be the culprits. Evolution tells us that animal fats are much more natural than vegetable oils. Human beings have been eating animal fats for millions of years. By now the digestive system and arteries should be completely adapted to this substance. Vegetable fats, on the other hand, are usually derived by squeezing seeds to extract their oil. This is a historically recent food-processing technique, and our digestive systems have had little time to adapt to vegetable oils. Some oils in wide use, such as peanut and cotton-seed oil, are brand new. The cotton seed has never been a natural food of man. Even corn was only introduced to the diets of Europeans several centuries ago, when maize was discovered in Central America. Compared to animal fats, corn oil is also a new substance.

The revolution in the reduction of dietary fiber and the increased consumption of refined carbohydrates began in the late 1800s. The epidemic of coronary artery disease appears to be similarly recent. If we implicate fat as a cause of coronary artery disease, there should have been an increase in the intake of fat, but this is not the case. On the contrary, fat consumption has increased little compared to the enormous decrease in fiber and increase in refined carbohydrate consumption.

While there are many studies of fiber that tell the story clearly, comparative studies that include Americans are very rare. The best of these compared Irish men who emigrated to the United States with their familial brothers who remained in Ireland. There were 1,154 subjects in this study. Half were in Boston, Massachusetts, and the other half in Ireland.

Even the background data on these two groups is revealing. Electrocardiograph studies indicated that the men in Boston had twice the rate of coronary artery disease as their brothers in Ireland. Also, 29 percent of all deaths of these men in Ireland in the forty-five to sixty-four-year age group were from coronary disease, whereas 42 percent of all deaths in second generation Irish-Americans in Massachusetts were due to coronary disease.

The Boston men had higher blood cholesterol than their Irish brothers. This was true even though the diet of the Irish men was somewhat higher in fat, particularly in animal fat. It was the

Boston brothers who ate the most polyunsaturated vegetable fats and the least animal fat. We would have expected, at least from what is generally proclaimed about eating animal fats and vegetable fats, that the Irish brothers would have had higher blood cholesterol, but they did not. The Irish ate more animal fats and had lower cholesterol.

Since these brothers spent their formative childhood years together, quite a number of factors were similar. These included the intake of protein, cholesterol, cigarette smoking, alcohol consumption, and blood pressures. Their intake of sugar was also alike. The Irish men ate an average of 3,768 calories a day, whereas their Boston brothers ate an average of 3,075 calories. Included in this 700-calorie-a-day difference was a considerably higher starch intake by the Irish brothers. They ate 267 grams of starch a day as opposed to the Boston men, who ate 116 grams of starch a day.

It is the difference in their fiber intake that tells the story. The Irish brothers ate an average of 6.4 grams of fiber a day, whereas those in Boston ate an average of 3.6 grams a day. Furthermore, the fiber in the diet of the Irish men came mostly from cereals and grains, whereas in Boston it was derived primarily from fruits and vegetables. This confirms other findings, both in humans and animals, that indicate that the fiber derived from cereal products is much more protective against coronary artery disease than the fiber derived from fruits and vegetables.

So here again is one of those amazing contradictions. The group that ate the most animal fat had the lower blood cholesterol. The group that had the higher calorie and starch intake had half the amount of heart disease as the other group.

Only one factor can account for this striking difference in the rates of coronary artery disease between these two groups of brothers—fiber.

The study of the Boston-Irish brothers parallels other studies of groups who eat large amounts of fiber and little refined carbohydrates. In fact, just because the Irish brothers have a lower incidence of coronary artery disease does not mean that they should stop there. They have certainly not reached the low-level of heart disease of the high-fiber African societies. If the Irish men wanted to reduce their risk of coronary artery disease even further, they should eat more fiber, just as I advise Americans to do.

My goal is to make practical use of the evidence these high-fiber eating societies provide us. Our society has a high incidence of coronary artery disease. Other groups have a lower incidence; in some their incidence is nearly zero. Hopefully, you will follow my recommendations in later chapters and help make coronary artery disease nearly nonexistent in America as well.

There is a controversy concerning fiber and sugar that I must report to you. Dr. John Yudkin is a distinguished British medical researcher who has for years advocated banning sugar from human consumption. He presents evidence that it is the intake of sugar that matches the occurrence of coronary disease around the world. If you read the findings of Yudkin and compare them with studies that indicate that fiber deficiency is the cause of coronary artery disease, you begin to realize that there is a correspondence between the decreased intake of fiber and the increased intake of refined sugar. You begin to see that these views are probably consistent with each other.

Why do sugar and fiber correlate so well? Societies that are more primitive generally have a higher fiber intake, and they also eat very little refined sugar. Our affluent Western societies have a low fiber intake and a high sugar intake. When a society moves from poverty to affluence, it generally takes one to three decades for its eating habits to change. During this period of change people usually begin reducing their consumption of fiber and start eating more refined sugar. There are very few societies which do one of these alone, and the evidence from them can often be used to support either a fiber deficiency cause or an excess consumption of refined sugar cause.

Which of these two factors, sugar or fiber, is more responsible? It is too early to say, though it is quite possible that both act together to cause coronary disease. The cause might be the combined absence of fiber and the high intake of refined sugar.

PEPTIC ULCER

The incidence of peptic ulcer is on the increase. It was actually a rare disease in the 1800s. Why is it more common today?

Many believe that ulcers are caused by stress, but is this true? Is today's busy executive under more stress than members of the tiny Stone-Age tribe, huddling in caves by night, fearful of predatory animals by day? Wasn't there considerable stress in medieval Europe, when brigands freely roamed the countryside and lords built huge castles for protection from one another, when peasant serfs had to leave their huts to till their lord's fields and then scurry back at dusk, often afraid that their own lord would prove a greater thief than the robber on the highways?

In the 1800s, when peptic ulcers were rare, there was great stress in the factories of the Industrial Revolution, where child and adult workers toiled long days for meager wages, while robber barons battled each other for control of huge trusts.

Yet it is today that peptic ulcers have grown common, even though stress has obviously been a constant part of human life since its beginnings. Today in England 10 percent of the male and 4 percent of the female population have clinically diagnosed ulcers at some time during their lives. And autopsies show that ulcers are suffered by about 20 percent of the population, regardless of sex.

What has changed? What might be the real cause of peptic ulcers today?

The current explanation suggests there is an internal battle between several substances secreted by the stomach wall. On the one side, hydrochloric acid and pepsin aid in the digestion of food. On the other side, mucin coats the stomach wall and protects it from being digested. If the amount of acid and pepsin increases and disturbs the acid-pepsin/mucin ratio, the stomach becomes vulnerable to attack from its own secretions.

Yet peptic ulcers are almost completely absent in some parts of the world. In fact, the incidence of peptic ulcer follows the intake of refined carbohydrates and is rare in high-fiber eating groups. At the Charles Johnson Memorial Hospital in Nqutu, South Africa, in the ten-year period from 1950 to 1960, only two cases of peptic ulcer were found out of 25,000 patients. The people in this area eat, for the most part, unrefined corn.

A report from a government radiologist in rural Ethiopia indicates that the incidence of peptic ulcer is 2 out of 1,000 patients, and that generally speaking, these 2 cases can be traced to the subject's eating Westernized foods. Yet in the large towns of Ethiopia, such as Addis Ababa, where there is plenty of white flour and white sugar, there is a great deal of peptic ulcer.

A report from the Wusasa Hospital in Nigeria, where something known as guinea corn is the chief food, states that in twelve years only 2 cases of peptic ulcer were seen. These people were all black.

But in the United States Army, peptic ulcer was shown to be as common in blacks as in whites.

Until the early part of this century, peptic ulcer was uncommon among blacks in the United States. This was at a time when a major item in the diet of black people was hominy, made from unrefined corn.

In societies that eat rice, those groups that eat hand-pounded rice have practically no peptic ulcers. Those groups that eat milled rice show a high incidence. Forty-five years ago autopsies in Sumatra on 1,370 Chinese immigrants showed 151 ulcers or evidence of past ulcer. Autopsies of 1,300 Javanese men living there showed only 8 ulcers. At that time the Chinese immigrants ate milled rice but the Javanese ate hand-pounded rice.

During this same time, in China, where hand-pounded rice was eaten, peptic ulcer was rare.

The incidence of peptic ulcer varies throughout India. It shows a direct correlation to the eating of milled rice as compared to those regions where hand-pounded rice is eaten.

The country with the highest incidence of peptic ulcer is Japan. The most common diet there is milled rice, and great quantities of refined sugar are consumed.

This worldwide evidence shows that peptic ulcers occur almost exclusively when the right dietary factors are present, factors that are not compatible with the normal functioning of the digestive system. Researchers do not know for certain whether there is an individual predisposition for peptic ulcers, but this recent research suggests to me that a certain percentage of the population will suffer these ulcers when the society has removed fiber from the diet and consumes sufficient amounts of refined carbohydrates.

This evidence indicates that the mechanism that causes the start of an ulcer is the removal of the natural buffering agents contained in food. In other words, the stomach's secretion of mucin is not the only device that protects against the hydrochloric acid and pepsin. Food offers protection also.

But it is only protein that neutralizes acid and pepsin. Fats, starches, and sugars do not have this effect.

During the refining of carbohydrates, protein is stripped from the carbohydrate. For example, in the extraction of sugar from the sugar beet, 100 percent of the protein is removed. In the milling of whole wheat, 11.2 percent of the original protein is removed. In the milling of rice, 30 percent of the protein is removed. And in the peeling and boiling of potatoes, between 4 and 16 percent of the protein is lost. Overconsumption of these protein-stripped foods tends to displace the intake of other foods that might contain protein, thus further reducing the protein intake.

Imagine going to the movies and eating a box of candy. The movie lasts for two hours. The candy puts practically pure sugar into your stomach. This stimulates the secretion of hydrochloric acid, and your stomach's lining is exposed for hours to virtually pure acid with absolutely no protein to help neutralize it.

Another finding might help explain the development of ulcers in single, isolated sites within the stomach. X-ray studies tend to show that eating different foods one at a time produces a layering effect of the foods in the stomach. The meal is not churned into one homogeneous mass. As a result, the lining of the stomach may be exposed to concentrated zones of acid without much buffering effect.

Dr. Cleave believes that the inconsistent eating of protein explains the source of ulcers. Even though we eat large amounts of protein with dinner, usually with lunch, and many times with breakfast, we also eat frequent between-meal snacks. Many people also eat super-refined and sugared cereal for breakfast, and sometimes a sandwich with little protein in it or only a salad for lunch. At those snacks and meals that do not contain animal protein we are consuming plant foods which, if unrefined, would contain more protein and provide a greater buffering effect. Since we have refined these foods, the calories are stripped naked and they offer very little protection.

This belief was reinforced in 1968, when the medical journal *Gut* reported an experiment in which the stomach's acidity increased after eating refined grain more than it did after eating unrefined grains.

Perhaps the most dramatic evidence comes from Americans taken prisoner by the Japanese in World War II, as reported by Dr. Cleave. In Singapore and Thailand the diet in the prisoner-of-war camps was milled rice. However, it was "supplemented" by rice polishings—the stripped "bran" of rice, which is high in fiber. Peptic ulcer was very infrequent. At the end of 1943 the rice polishings were discontinued, and in 1944 duodenal ulcer became rampant.

In 1943 the Japanese took large numbers of prisoners from Singapore to Thailand to work on the Burma railway. By the time they returned to Singapore in 1944, 40 percent had died from the horrible conditions to which they were exposed.

Strangely enough, in the midst of this unbelievable stress where four out of ten prisoners died, peptic ulcer was rare. Why? Their diet was supplemented by rice bran, which was usually fed to pigs.

Prisoners in Hong Kong suffered greatly from peptic ulcer, on a diet consisting mainly of milled rice. However, at one point many were transferred to Japan, and their diet was changed to a mixture that included unmilled grains. The incidence of ulcers was reduced to virtually zero.

In Tokyo, over a one-year period, there wasn't a single case reported among 6,000 prisoners; and in Cobia and Osaka, only one case was reported among 7,000 to 8,000 prisoners. The native Japanese, of course, with their milled rice diet, had a very high incidence.

The argument that stress is the main factor is refuted by these various studies of prisoner-of-war camps, where stress must have been considerable.

The other theaters of World War II provided more information on peptic ulcers. It is a well-known fact that they were very common in the German Army. Peptic ulcers were so common that whole units of soldiers, as a group, were put on ulcer diets.

An interesting study comes from the German soldiers who fought at the Russian front during the bitter winter of 1943. The farther the front lines got from Germany, the more the German soldiers were cut off from their supply lines. Many of them were forced to pick raw potatoes, turnips, and other vegetables and eat them straight from the ground. Some were fortunate enough to eat grains left behind by the Russians. These grains were eaten completely unprocessed. The incidence of peptic ulcer dropped dramatically among these soldiers.

After the war, 2,000 repatriated Germans who had been Russian prisoners showed virtually no ulcer symptoms from their years in captivity. Yet they suffered a complete reversal on their return to Germany, with its refined carbohydrates, sugars, and sweets.

Why were ulcers rare in the 1800s? Why are they common

today? The refining of grain and sugar started in the late 1800s. Today, societies that still eat unrefined foods have a very low ulcer incidence. Even war prisoners, who suffered stress but were protected by the unrefined "bran" of rice, had a low incidence. Now isn't the answer clear?

TOOTH DECAY

Tooth decay is a much more serious health problem than it might appear at first glance. This minute it may have an aura of less then critical importance. But think how you feel when you are lying back in your dentist's chair, squinting against the bright, blinding light, trying to ignore the whine of the drill and the menacing shape of the teeth-pulling pliers, feeling less than reassured by his or her chatter, and anxious because the bill will upset your month's budget.

For our society as a whole, tooth decay and gum disease are almost frightening dental problems. Hundreds of millions of cavities are filled each year. There is a backlog of over a billion unfilled cavities. Millions of Americans wear false teeth because of both tooth decay and gum disease.

This ailment can be studied statistically and epidemiologically, comparing societies with different kinds of diets. The dental remains from ancient peoples have also been scrutinized, and they have yielded valuable secrets about humanity's changing eating habits.

Can tooth decay actually be increased or reduced by the kinds of foods we eat? Many prominent authorities agree with this idea in their widely quoted dictum, "Avoid sweets between meals." But I go beyond this to another proposition, that additional fiber and the reduction of refined carbohydrates can increase the health of both your teeth and your gums.

There is a difference between the location of dental decay in our refined-food age as compared to ancient peoples. Studies done on recovered skulls indicate that in ancient peoples tooth decay was present mainly beneath the gum line. Particles of food were probably driven beneath the gum where bacterial growth produced chemicals that ate into the tooth. Today we see dental caries higher on the teeth, on the enamel, where it should be very difficult for food to become trapped. If the offender were sugar alone, it would be almost impossible for it to remain on the rather smooth enamel surfaces where most of today's tooth decay occurs.

Dr. Cleave clearly states in his book that he believes tooth decay is caused by the consumption of refined carbohydrates. He believes that it is the refining of flour and the refining of sugar that contributes to our high rates of tooth decay.

When sugar is combined with the rather sticky refined flour (and almost all commercial breads are made with sugar), it produces a very adhering glue that plasters itself to the enamel surfaces. Bacterial growth then proceeds, producing acids that attack the teeth. It is the sticky quality of refined white flour that makes it so desirable for bread-making and inclusion in other foods, but that also creates the paste that helps foster tooth decay.

When we compare our diet of processed white bread with the rice diets of Oriental cultures, we note an immediate and obvious difference. Refined rice does not have this sticky quality, and rice-eating cultures have a very low incidence of tooth decay.

As we delve further into the epidemiological evidence, other interesting cases await our discovery. One case is from an island called Tristan da Cunha in the remote southern Atlantic Ocean. In 1932, consistent with the introduction of refined carbohydrates to the island, the population experienced a sudden deterioration of the teeth.

Some extremely serious periodontal diseases may also result from eating refined carbohydrates and eliminating fiber from our diets. Chewing rough, coarse, and fibrous foods helps keep the gums hard and keritinized. Fiber itself does not prevent diseases of the gums, but the frequent eating, and therefore chewing, of fibrous foods should stimulate the gums and help prevent gum disease.

DIABETES

Diabetes afflicts millions in our country. It is unquestionably a very serious, sometimes lethal disease. There is a split in opinion among American doctors as to whether or not diet is a causative factor. But the split in opinion is not mirrored by the evidence seen when we leave the laboratory and compare societies who eat high-fiber diets with our own. There, the evidence is clear: diet does appear to play a significant role in the existence of diabetes.

In most countries, coronary disease is commonly associated with diabetes. Where one is present, the other is also found. Where coronary disease is rare, diabetes is also rare.

Though medical science leaps ahead with striking new techniques such as kidney transplants, in theoretical areas it is very conservative. The medical community is slow to accept new theories; often this is a good attitude, because the application of new theories sometimes produces unexpected problems. But in some cases this attitude works against the health of the public, and people suffer needlessly from disease because the medical community is reluctant to consider large bodies of carefully researched data.

If a doctor were to state categorically that diabetes is caused by the overconsumption of sugar, he would be met with a barrage of criticism. Well-guarded and carefully worded statements, such as by Dr. John Yudkin, a British scientist, are indeed very daring. He states that, "eating too much sugar is one of the reasons why people get diabetes." And then, in his book *Sweet and Dangerous,* he goes on to present almost incontrovertible evidence to support his belief.

Dr. Cleave has proposed a biological mechanism that makes a good deal of sense to me. The pancreas is the gland that secretes the hormone insulin, which is responsible for regulating the amount of sugar in the blood. The pancreas becomes strained from overwork when the habitual intake of normal amounts of refined sugar becomes excessive. This strain on the pancreas causes it to malfunction. Of course, this only occurs in a small percentage of the population, and this is the group that develops diabetes.

Refined sugar surges into the bloodstream far more rapidly than unrefined sugar that is still in its natural state. Furthermore, overconsumption of sugar and of carbohydrates occurs as a result of the body's being deceived in its perception of what it has consumed.

The average American consumes just over four ounces of refined sugar a day—in sodas, candy, cakes, ice cream, doughnuts, or other sweets. This consumption takes a minimum of effort, and the foods do little to satisfy the appetite. The refining process has deceived your body, which has no way of judging the large quantity of calories it has really taken in.

You would have to eat two and a half pounds of sugar beets to consume the same four ounces of sugar in its natural state. Or you would have to eat approximately twenty apples. It is unlikely that anyone would eat either of these. Should any of us accomplish this, we would not want to eat anything else—as we regularly do when we consume sweets, adding two scoops of vanilla ice cream to our slice of apple pie, or an extra doughnut to our morning coffee break.

The epidemiological evidence is overwhelming. In Natal, South Africa, there is a group of Indians who are descendants of a smaller group that emigrated from India. The average yearly sugar intake of these African Indians is over 110 pounds per person. Their relatives in India eat between 12 and 15 pounds of sugar a year. The incidence of diabetes in these 400,000 African Indians is quite high compared to those in India. Furthermore, the incidence of diabetes in these African Indians is much higher than in the tribal Zulus who live in the same area, but who consume very little refined sugar.

Further evidence comes from within India itself. In southern India the diet consists mainly of milled white rice, but little sugar. There the incidence of diabetes is high. The white rice contains carbohydrates in the form of starch, which is readily converted to sugar in the digestive tract and bloodstream. In northern India the diet consists mainly of unrefined wheat and corn. Both the wheat and corn contain starch, but they are also high in fiber—and the incidence of diabetes is quite low.

In a test of 2,000 sugarcane cutters in Africa, only three had urine that contained even a trace of sugar. From a medical standpoint, this is an extremely low percentage, considering the amount of sugarcane they eat. While sugarcane is extremely high in calories and sugar, it is also extremely high in fiber. This is another piece of the epidemiological puzzle that suggests that fibrous food protects us while fiber-free food does not.

A very similar finding was reported by Dr. Frederick Banting, who received the Nobel Prize for his contribution to the discovery of insulin. In 1924 he observed that of 5,000 native workers who applied for work in the construction of the Panama Canal, only two were found who had sugar in their urine. These people were natives and one of their main food items was sugarcane. Wealthy Spaniards in the same region ate large quantities of refined sugar and had a very high incidence of diabetes.

An Israeli scientist, Dr. A. M. Cohen, presented a revealing comparative study. Jews generally suffer from a very high incidence of diabetes. Dr. Cohen compared Jews who emigrated to Israel from four different backgrounds: the Western world, North Africa, recent arrivals from Yemen, and those who had emigrated from Yemen some twenty years before. The only group that had a low incidence of diabetes were the recent arrivals from Yemen. All of the others, including the Yemenites who had arrived twenty years before, had approximately the same proportion of diabetes. The major difference in the diet of the two Yemenite groups was that, after coming to Israel, the earlier group had greatly increased its consumption of sugar. This earlier group was rewarded for its high sugar intake by a rate of diabetes fifty times that of its newly arrived countrymen.

What about urban Africans, those who live in the cities of Africa and eat a refined carbohydrate diet closer to our own? They have the same incidence of diabetes as American blacks. And American blacks have about the same incidence as American whites.

Epidemiological evidence pours in from all over the globe. Canadian Eskimos have recently started eating large amounts of sugar, and diabetes among them is climbing rapidly. Eskimos in Greenland do not eat refined sugar, and they have very little diabetes.

Studies done in Trinidad showed a lower incidence among the black inhabitants than among the East Indian inhabitants. Here, both groups ate a considerable amount of sugar daily. The dietary difference that could account for the lower rate of diabetes among the blacks was that they consumed a larger proportion of fiber in the form of unrefined cereals.

In Iceland a hundred years ago diabetes was virtually unknown and so was refined sugar. Today a high consumption of refined sugar is accompanied by a high incidence of diabetes.

There is a great deal more evidence available from all over the world. The conclusion seems unavoidable: the relationship between refined sugar, the absence of fiber, and diabetes can no longer be ignored.

CANCER OF THE COLON AND POLYPS OF THE COLON

Dr. Denis Burkitt was quoted in a 1972 issue of *Medical World News.* He expressed the opinion that a number of diseases may have a common cause. He went on to say that these diseases are cancer of the colon, diverticular disease, ulcerative colitis, polyps of the colon, and appendicitis. Then he named the suspected cause of these diseases: the absence of fiber in the diet.

When African blacks were first brought to this country, cancer of the colon was unknown among them. Today in Africa it accounts for only 2 percent of all cancers. Have the American blacks escaped this disease by some hereditary strength in their bodies? No—today American blacks suffer cancer of the colon equal to whites.

In the United States cancer of the colon is the most common cancer, striking even more people than lung cancer. However, cancer of the colon is only the second-biggest killer, as lung cancer claims more lives. The state of Connecticut has the unfortunate distinction of having the highest incidence of cancer of the colon in the world.

The mechanism believed to cause cancer of the colon starts with the growth of bacteria in the stool as it passes through the digestive system. These bacteria decompose bile salts and produce new chemicals that have been shown to be potentially carcinogenic, or cancer causing. The bile salts come from the bile, the secretion of the gall bladder that aids in the digestion of fats. This bile then passes through the digestive tract and is eliminated with the feces.

On a low-fiber diet food travels abnormally slowly through the digestive system. Because of the extended travel time, these bacteria multiply and produce larger quantities of carcinogens than when the food is moving quickly. The low-fiber diet also gives these carcinogens more time to remain in direct contact with the mucosa of the colon, where they may cause cancer.

In addition, the low-fiber stool is smaller in volume, so the carcinogens produced by bile decomposition turn out to be a more concentrated chemical working on each individual area of the colon for a longer time.

Experimental work on animals supports this mechanism. In one experiment the terminal portion of the colon was bypassed, so that no feces passed through it. When this was done, no cancers developed in the colon. This implicates a substance in the feces as the causative agent.

Like other cancers, colon-rectum cancer can be cured if it is caught at an early stage. But the examination for early detection is only rarely used—because a half-inch-thick flexible colonscope that examines all six feet of your large intestine for 30 minutes, without anesthesia, is not a comfortable or an inexpensive procedure. As in all the naked calorie diseases, the best cure is prevention.

I won't burden you with endless statistics. Similar examples could be repeated over and over again. I will just point out that those groups of people who have higher levels of fiber in their diet also have a low rate of cancer of the colon.

Polyps of the colon, which are a noncancerous growth, affect 20 percent of the adult population of the United States, but are scarcely to be found among Africans. A small percentage of these polyps—estimates range as high as 7 percent—eventually become cancerous.

These diseases, cancer of the colon and polyps of the colon, are virtually unknown among animals that eat natural diets. There is one exception, however. The domestic dogs of industrialized countries who eat human leftovers also suffer from these ailments.

In coming chapters I will introduce a diet that might not only substantially reduce your chances of getting cancer of the colon, but may help protect you from suffering any of the diseases discussed here.

GALLSTONES, APPENDICITIS, AND OTHER DISEASES

Researchers have noted that the presence of fiber in the diet seems to protect against the development of gallstones. Epidemiological evidence is available. The final verdict as to whether or not gallstones are caused by a deficiency of fiber in the diet is not yet in because the mechanism that is suggested is so complicated.

I have already briefly mentioned appendicitis and its relationship to a low-fiber diet. Both appendicitis and gallstones exist primarily in the industrialized Western world, where food is processed and refined. Both are virtually nonexistent in developing countries where high-fiber diets are eaten.

Researchers have suggested that a number of other ailments are caused by these same factors, either by the removal of fiber, by the increased consumption of refined carbohydrates, or both. Among these ailments is hiatus hernia, which occurs when the upper portion of the stomach pushes its way through the diaphragm into the chest cavity. It is even possible that high blood pressure and gout are related to a processed diet.

If the naked calorie is responsible for the impressive list of diseases covered in this chapter, and if it causes widespread medical havoc in our society, is it likely that we have discovered the full extent of this epidemic? These revelations are fairly recent and have only been observed and studied by a relatively small number of doctors. It seems logical to assume that there will be new connections discovered between the naked calorie and other diseases, connections that we don't even dream exist.

For instance, one researcher is studying the possibility that the carcinogens formed by bacterial decomposition of bile salts (see the section on cancer of the colon) may be absorbed by the mucosa of the colon and transported to other parts of the body, where they may cause some forms of cancer, such as breast cancer.

It seems likely that the views of medical science on the causes and treatment of a multitude of ailments are about to change substantially. As a result of this change, we may become a much healthier society. The groundwork has been laid, and this book shows you the tremendous distance that has already been covered. Let us hope that our professional health specialists seek a healthier future with determination, and sweep over all the obstacles that may confront them.

There is an immediate opportunity for you to improve your

health now that you have learned of these findings. You and I do not have to wait for the stream of explanations that medical researchers will develop over the next ten or twenty years. We can act now. We already know an astonishing list of diseases and ailments that are related to the naked calorie. Let us have no more naked calories!

Perhaps we can rid ourselves of a major cause of many diseases. Perhaps this time we will lose our excess pounds and learn to maintain our proper weight easily!

HIGH-FIBER PROTECTION

When I discussed cancer of the colon, I suggested how fiber protects the lower intestine from carcinogenic chemicals produced by bacteria. Fiber speeds these cancer-causing chemicals through the intestine faster than they can cause damage, and ties them up in its bulk so they are eliminated in the feces.

This bodily protection is an important benefit from a high-fiber diet, and Dr. Benjamin Ershoff has produced additional evidence supporting this. The processed foods from our technologically based food industry subject us to a host of chemical food additives, insecticides, preservatives, dyes, and other ingredients, most of which have never been thoroughly tested.

In a series of experiments Dr. Ershoff fed two diets to several paired groups of laboratory mice. One group was fed a diet high in fiber. The other group's diet was fiber-free. Then he fed each of these paired groups an additional harmful chemical along with their diet.

In one experiment he fed a paired group the common food additive Tween 60, which is an emulsifying agent. The Tween 60 proved lethal to the fiber-free group when greater than 5 percent of the diet, but the same amount of the chemical did not produce any ill effects in the group on a high-fiber diet.

Ershoff tested two other common food additives (red dye #2 and sodium cyclamate) and a drug (chlorazanil hydrochloride);

they produced ill effects in the mice fed a fiber-free diet, but were either tolerable or harmless in the group fed the high-fiber diet.

Some of the physical illnesses we suffer may come from one or more of the chemicals or insecticides we consume in our food. In fact, the estimated annual consumption of these chemicals is four pounds per person, a considerable amount. Yet if the evidence on laboratory animals holds true for human beings, fiber in the diet may protect us against the ill effects of the chemicals we eat, in the same way that it protects us from the cancerous toxins produced by bacteria in our intestines.

STOPPING THE NAKED CALORIE DISEASE

As you have seen, evidence on an astonishing number of serious diseases and common ailments is pouring in from around the world. Researchers in many countries are hard at work. Amazingly enough, they are frequently searching for proof that these diseases do not exist in a particular society, primarily in those groups who eat high-fiber diets. Who would have thought that the most valuable medical data would turn out to be proof that a society was not afflicted by a particular disease?

But this is the evidence that reveals that our own raging epidemic of these diseases may be unnecessary. And this discovery may prove as important in improving your health as the breakthrough development of antibiotics has been during the last thirty-five years.

Coronary artery disease, cancer of the colon, diabetes, peptic ulcers, diverticular disease, and the rest are all manifestations of a single epidemic—which I have named the Naked Calorie Disease.

Most striking of all, it is an environmental disease. It is not caused by a bug, such as tuberculosis or influenza—although it strikes and kills so many people you probably agree that it is as important to conquer as tuberculosis itself. In fact, eliminating the Naked Calorie Disease could be an important victory in the war on cancer, because it might help to knock out the second most murderous form of cancer.

We are at the threshold of a new kind of treatment for this huge medical problem, this environmental epidemic. Its cause is found in the food we eat, and, by making two simple changes in our diet, we can effectively reduce our risk of contracting many diseases, and perhaps rid our society of the whole Naked Calorie Disease. Until we make these two dietary changes, eating our usual meals will be like breathing the polluted air from automobile exhaust.

When our society realized the danger that air pollution caused, an Environmental Protection Agency was set up to mandate rules to reduce the poisons manufacturers were permitted to spew into the air. We must work from the ground up to build a social mandate to (1) add fiber to our diets, and (2) eliminate the intake of refined carbohydrates, sugar, and white flour. That is the path to greater health and well being.

As you come to the fork in your own path and weigh your choices, it may help if you remember how the poet Robert Frost once decided which path was best for him to follow: ". . . I chose the one less traveled by, and that made all the difference." In the same way that the poet chooses the path that opens to him the best life can offer, you can choose the best gift you can give your body—health.

None of the subdiseases that are manifestations of the Naked Calorie Disease springs into existence overnight. Every one is an environmentally caused disease. It takes years, sometimes decades, of dietary stresses and strains to produce such a disease. Some, like tooth decay, can be started in a matter of months. Others, like peptic ulcer, can arise in less than a few years. But most of them, like coronary artery disease, cancer of the colon, and diverticulitis need many years of incubation.

Studies of smokers who have quit show their lungs soon begin to lose their filthy, gray accumulation of grime and return to their natural, healthy pink state within six to nine months after quitting. In fact, statistical studies show that someone who quits smoking nearly eliminates his or her chances for contracting lung cancer.

We do not yet have studies that show the recovery rate of people who have begun eating high-fiber diets and have eliminated refined carbohydrates. But we do know that the human body has remarkable recuperative powers, and, given half a chance, will generally come through and return to full health.

The aim of this book is to interrupt and end the incubation of the diseases caused by the lack of fiber in the diet. These diseases grow and form inside us for decades. As the study of smokers has already proved, and I am certain that future statistics will bear me out: once you have ended the incubation of these diseases in your body, you will return to health and well being. Your body's natural systems of immunity to disease will work better, and your chances of contracting these diseases will be substantially reduced.

Your war with the Naked Calorie Disease will have been won.

CHAPTER 4

SHOULD WE RELY ON EPIDEMIOLOGICAL EVIDENCE?

The medical breakthrough on the importance of fiber in the diet is a classic case of the use of epidemiological evidence. Quite a number of important medical discoveries begin this way. As happened in South Africa with the Zulus, a doctor observes that a certain group of people exhibit the common presence or absence of a particular ailment. He or she searches for the common factor responsible for this. Sometimes it is obvious; other times it is very difficult to discover.

Once this causative or protective agent is discovered, the usual next step is to test it and develop experimental evidence. Two experimental groups are selected. This agent is administered to one group and omitted from the other. The results of the experiment either confirm or deny what the doctor suspected.

In the case of the diseases I have mentioned, there is a great deal of epidemiological evidence to support my belief that increased dietary fiber could greatly decrease the occurrence of certain diseases. Now we should experiment with groups of volunteers, feeding some high-fiber diets and others our regular Western diet. We could meticulously record their intakes and periodically examine them for evidence of disease. But, as we have seen, the suspected incubation periods for many of these ailments can be twenty, thirty, or even forty years. Even if we could find volunteers sufficiently dedicated to complete these experiments, the benefits derived could only be enjoyed by those born twenty, thirty, or forty years in the future.

What about the millions who are now in the process of acquiring these ailments? Shall doctors abandon any effort to help them because this experiment has not yet been performed?

Actually, it could be argued that this experiment has been performed in the reverse in other countries. Former high-fiber eating societies that have adopted our refined food diet have experienced a rise in these diseases twenty, thirty, and forty years after they have made this change.

This same occurrence can be seen in our society, beginning about a hundred years ago. Our hospitals and our medical research laboratories see the results of it today, as they struggle to heal these illnesses and discover new cures. You yourself see its results, because you carry excess pounds that you have not been able to shed.

Since my diet involves good, plain, natural food and not experimental drugs with their potential for unknown side effects, there seems little reason to wait three decades while a long and slow medical experiment is carried out. This experiment will certainly be done. If the obvious is eventually fully corroborated, then we have all benefitted by following the extremely strong epidemiological evidence I have presented. If the benefits are less than I anticipate, we have suffered no harm in the attempt, and we may have received at least one benefit: the reduction of obesity and the control of weight.

Some people may want to understand more about what epidemiological evidence is. In Appendix A I present a mythical example of this kind of evidence, where it comes from, and what it teaches us.

But for those of you who this minute are more concerned about your weight, the next chapter begins to explain how to add fiber to your diet, and how it will work to control your weight.

CHAPTER 5

THE REBIRTH OF YOUR DIGESTIVE SYSTEM

You have seen how the absence of fiber in the diet combined with the consumption of refined foods can lead to obesity and impaired health in Americans, as well as in other peoples who have made the transition to "modern" diets. You have also followed the introduction of refined foods into our own society. By now you have probably guessed that I shall advocate the reintroduction of this missing fiber into our diets. You are indeed correct, and this will be the cornerstone of my program for achieving and maintaining a sensible weight.

While I have treated tens of thousands of patients for weight problems, I cannot personally hope to reach even a tiny percentage of the millions afflicted with obesity and the epidemic I have called the Naked Calorie Disease. My hope is that this book will aid those millions who need help.

Helping to build a society of healthier, sensible-eating adults and children is my goal. Admittedly, this goal is an ideal, but it is also a potential social movement that could directly benefit millions of Americans. In fact, the health benefits derived from my proposed diet may render the obesity problem a minor one, if obesity could ever be called "minor." In the same way that a vaccination protects you from smallpox or polio before you develop the disease, you no longer have to wait to become ill to begin combatting the naked calorie diseases. They have an incubation period. They are developing in you right now. But you can stop the process by improving your diet immediately.

When our society discovers that we are drinking cancer-causing asbestos in our water or breathing it in the air, we act to remove this mineral from contact with us. Why shouldn't we do the same with our diets, removing what are most likely disease-causing elements and adding the healthier foods it lacks?

Obviously, not all of us will start eating sensibly, even if doing so were guaranteed to prolong our lives. Too many people are conditioned to eating poorly at every meal. When they get to the office in the morning, doughnuts and coffee, with an extra teaspoonful of refined sugar, is the bad habit that chains millions of stomachs to improper digestion. Rich cakes, pies, and ice cream for dessert every night shocks their digestive systems even more. White bread in their sandwiches, excessively fat-laden luncheon meats, and vitamin-drained vegetables all do their share to bring their health to a lower ebb than it should be.

The Surgeon General's famous report on smoking and health exploded on the scene in 1964, but it did little to change the smoking habits of many Americans. Yet many were helped, and millions have quit smoking since that date. Indeed, many more will quit, as they arrive at their doctor's office complaining of chest pains, hacking coughs, and shortened breath, only to discover that the years of self-inflicted abuse have finally taken their toll. "Stop smoking immediately!" will be the edict. Since their addiction will become a matter of life or death, most of them will finally stop smoking.

All too often it will be too late. The damage will have been done. The weakened lungs through which they must gasp for breath, and the weakened heart that cannot afford to take a moment's rest will be up against the thin edge of their diminished capabilities.

It has been discovered that the surest way to stop people from smoking is for a doctor to sit them down, personally explain that smoking is killing them, explain to them the consequences they will suffer, and then forcefully order them to give up this habit. If this is the best way to stop a person from smoking, then perhaps the same procedure will work with your diet, another accumulation of bad habits that similarly threatens your life.

As a physician I have studied and treated obesity for many years, helping thousands of patients solve their problems. But now, major new findings point the way to better health in addition to easily maintaining your proper weight. Based on this new information I am going to personally give you my recommendation for the safest and most effective way to safeguard your health. I am going to explain the changes you will need to make in your diet, why you should begin changing your diet *immediately,* and how you can make this change with a minimum of difficulty and with *maximum results.*

Were I to see you personally in my office, we would sit down together and I would answer all your questions. I would explain to you the voluminous scientific data I have before me. I am sure you would soon be convinced. But you and I both know it is impossible for me to have this discussion with each of you. Instead, I will offer you this same, life-saving information in this book, probably in greater detail than you would ever have the chance to hear it from me or any other doctor in person.

I am sure you will wind up as convinced as I am. Like smoking, your final choice of diet will be your own, and you will live—or die—with your decision.

The two major changes in your diet center around the introduction of fiber-containing foods and the reduction or elimination of those foods that contain little or no fiber. These changes will primarily be in the foods which are of *plant* origin. Meat, fish, and fowl also form a part of the diet, but the major changes in your diet will be concerned with the type of plant foods you eat.

When I speak of plant foods, I am including all those foods that originate in the ground, such as grains, fruits, vegetables, nuts, seeds, etc. I am therefore including those foods that are made in part or totally from these plant foods, such as bread, candy, orange juice, and peanut butter. These are also the carbohydrate foods; although there is some carbohydrate in food derived from animals, for the most part we receive our carbohydrates from plants.

As I mentioned before, wheat bran is the food that contains more fiber than almost any other food. We are fortunate in this, because it is easy to use as an inexpensive and early invisible supplement to the diet. I will amplify this discussion of bran later. For the moment, I am going to discuss fiber. But remember, when I talk about adding fiber to your diet, this fiber will usually be in the form of bran.

Earlier I mentioned that the carbohydrate content of the plant is contained within the cell, but that the outer cell walls of most plants are mainly a container made out of cellulose, indigestible to human beings. These cell walls, which I shall henceforth refer to simply as fiber, have no food value for the human body, yet they are still classified as carbohydrate. Therefore, food analysis charts (available by the hundreds all the way from the check-out counter of the supermarket to the medical library) will tell you the number of grams of carbohydrate in the various foods. But the values they list for carbohydrate include both the digestible carbohydrate and the indigestible fiber, which has no food value and which cannot possibly make you fat.

The situation is further confused by the fact that these charts list the calories for each food as the total number of calories contained in all the carbohydrate, including the indigestible portion. If these tables were to be corrected so that they gave the calorie content of only the carbohydrate *available* to us in digestible form, these values in general would appear lower than those now shown. The terms "available carbohydrate" and "unavailable carbohydrate" are terms regularly used by nutritional scientists.

What I'm trying to tell you is that when you look at charts and tables and add up the grams of carbohydrate you are eating, the amounts in your total are different from what your body actually receives. If your purpose is to try and find out how much carbohydrate is actually available to your body, then I'm afraid you are not succeeding. The tables aren't accurate!

I'm sure this is a shock to many of you. Some of you have used these tables for years and never suspected they weren't telling you the truth. Many of you have used these tables and been disappointed with the results you got. Something seemed to be "off," but you weren't sure what it was. The tables just didn't seem to be a satisfying way to figure out the food values you were receiving, because they didn't always appear to work consistently.

By how much are these tables incorrect? Since different plant foods have different amounts of fibrous content, those with the highest amounts of fiber have greater percentages of carbohydrates and calories unavailable. On the other hand, the carbohydrates and calories listed for those foods with the least amounts of fiber were nearly accurate. So your tables aren't consistently off. For some foods the tables are way off, and for other foods they are fairly accurate.

This is confusing to say the least, and as happens to so many of us, what confuses us discourages us, especially when we can't predict if something will or will not work. Charts and tables that combine accuracy, clarity, and direct usefulness are what the dieting public needs. But until the recent findings about fiber in foods, it was not possible to prepare them so that both the scientists and the dieting public would fully understand them and appreciate their value.

Where can you find tables that are right? Technically, the tables you now possess are accurate, but they won't solve your problem. What you need are tables that not only show the calories and the grams of carbohydrate, but also the amount of *fiber* contained in the food. Only in these new tables will you find the amounts of calories and carbohydrate that are actually *available* to your body from each food.

Can you buy these new tables? Sure—they're available in

medical books. But you'll have to do some calculating because you must consider the two crucial values, fiber and carbohydrate, in relation to one another.

If this sounds like a lot of work, and you're not very good in math, don't worry about it. I've done all the work for you. In Chapter 12 you will find tables that not only indicate the grams of carbohydrate and the number of calories but also the amount of crude fiber contained in the food. These tables accurately depict the actual amount of carbohydrate available to you. Even more important, you will find a new value given for each food. This is a new concept that I have developed, and it cannot be found anywhere else. It was invented to simplify your understanding of fiber, and make you successful in accomplishing a dietary change. I will soon tell you exactly what your dietary change will be, and the best ways you can accomplish it.

First you need to understand a little bit about how many calories your body actually receives from the foods you eat. Your present tables are incorrect because food contains varying amounts of fiber. When you eat fibrous foods your body actually "receives" fewer calories than you "eat." The calories that eventually find their way into your bloodstream are fewer than those that pass through your stomach and intestines. There are a number of factors that influence whether or not you receive all the calories you eat. The most important of these are (1) the form in which the food reaches your stomach; (2) the speed at which the food passes through your gastrointestinal tract; and, (3) the amount of dietary fiber contained in the food.

The form of the food influences how much of it is absorbed. For example, when you drink a glass of soda, which is essentially a solution of cane sugar in carbonated, flavored water, under most conditions your body receives an almost 100 percent absorption of the sugar. On the other hand, when you eat whole-kernel corn, which also contains a great deal of carbohydrate, you may absorb only a portion of its available carbohydrate. How well the food is chewed also influences absorption; you may have seen corn you did not chew well eliminated in a form very similar to that in which it entered your body. Here is a perfect example of a case where you ate and enjoyed a starchy, relatively high-calorie food but did not fully pay the price of added weight.

There is a clear difference between the weight you gain from drinking a glass of soda and eating an ear of corn if the corn is not fully chewed. Because the sugar is in a form that is easily absorbed, you receive all the calories in the soda. When you eat corn, you receive far less than the total number of calories it contains. Of course, I am not suggesting that you should chew some foods poorly. I am introducing the fact that there are ways to eat and enjoy foods, but that you do not have to gain additional weight at the same time.

Another factor that determines the amount of calories your body receives from the food you eat is the length of time this food is present in your digestive system. Since the weight you gain depends on the various digestive juices getting to and acting on the food you have swallowed, the length of time these juices have at their disposal influences how many calories you actually get out of the food. It takes time to completely digest every calorie. If you do not allow sufficient time to complete the digestion, your body will receive fewer calories. If food passes through at a sufficiently fast rate, there will not be time for all the food products to break down into a form that is absorbable. The number of calories you actually receive from food that travels through your body swiftly may be considerably less than that which the food actually contains.

How fast the food moves through your body is influenced by a number of factors. If you are suffering from diarrhea, the food passes through you at a very fast rate and only small amounts of calories are absorbed. This is, of course, an unpleasant way to lose weight, and severe dysentery can cause malnutrition and even, rarely, death by starvation. Other, less extreme factors that influence the speed of food through your body are your emotional state, the exercise you have had close to mealtime, and any drugs you have taken.

The introduction of fiber into the diet is another way to increase the speed at which food moves through your body. There is adequate medical evidence, based on studies of digestive rates in humans, to show that the transit time of food is greatly reduced when the diet is high in fiber.

This second factor in calorie absorption, the transit time of food in the body, brings us to the heart of the information that lies behind this book. I have just stated that the transit time of food is greatly reduced when the diet is high in dietary fiber. Now I am going to tell you that this is technically incorrect. What I should have said is that the transit time is *normal* with sufficient dietary fiber, for medical evidence shows this to be the normal diet intended for the human body. The transit time of our modern, ultra-refined, fiber-free diet is greatly prolonged.

As I said before, the human digestive system did not evolve amid urban conditions. Our digestive systems evolved to handle fiber because it was abundant in all the plant foods eaten since the dawn of humanity. Today we are only second- and third-generation processed-food eaters, because the removal of fiber only began in the late nineteenth century. Can we really expect our digestive systems to adapt this quickly to the vast changes we have made in the foods we eat? As disease and obesity evidence from around the world indicates, the normal human nutritional balance includes dietary fiber.

From this evidence, it appears that the diet that I recommend, part fiber and part available nutrients, is the proper diet for the human body. With this diet, the transit time of food through the body is shortened to its normal length when you ingest sufficient amounts of fiber with each meal. It is not that fibrous foods are laxatives, but rather that the refined foods you eat, the defibered foods, are constipating.

The modern, processed, fiber-free diet is the abnormal diet.

Its excess caloric and carbohydrate content prolongs its transit time through the body. Refined foods give you the worst of both worlds. The removal of fiber means that everything you eat is made of available calories and carbohydrates. And the resulting prolonged transit time means that you receive all the excess calories (and thus weight) refined food has to offer. You have your cake and you get fat from it too. Unquestionably, this fiber-free, processed-food diet is the main cause of obesity in our society.

I have seen the same drama enacted time after time. Individually, you formulate a serious intent: "It's time to lose some of that fat." Collectively, our medical authorities agree, "America needs to reduce its excess weight." But permanent weight loss is simply not possible for individuals or for millions of overweight Americans, when society compels them to continue eating a refined diet that forces extra pounds on them.

In practical terms, if you start eating foods high in dietary fiber you will notice an immediate change in your body. You can expect to have a bowel movement sooner than you would on your present diet. Generally, this does not mean that you will have more frequent bowel movements, although some of you may. It means that the food you eat will pass through you and leave your system much more quickly than it does on a refined diet.

This is a change for the better, for two reasons. First, it means that your body receives fewer calories because of the food's shorter transit time. You will begin to lose weight from this alone, or you will maintain your proper weight very easily. Second, it will point out to you the large difference between a diet of refined foods, and a diet that includes fiber. You will personally see that your body begins to "notice" this difference almost immediately.

An important benefit you will receive from dietary fiber is that you will bring your weight under control. The greater the percentage of fiber in the food you eat, the fewer calories your body will receive, and the faster you will lose weight. Therefore, when you diet to lose weight you will add more fiber to your meals. You will not only have fewer calories available, but the transit time of food through your body is reduced. You will eat enough to satisfy your hunger, yet the calories your body receives will be diminished.

Once you have reached the weight you want to maintain, the fiber in your diet will be adjusted to the proportion that will keep you at that weight without difficulty. The amount of fiber in your food will be adjusted individually, according to whether your purpose is weight maintenance or weight loss.

In addition to the factors that influence how many of the calories you eat are absorbed, other factors influence the quantity of food you actually ingest or eat. Here, the social situation in which you eat seems to be very important. For example, if you have a specific allotted lunch period and cannot prolong this time, you are limited by how much food you can stuff into your mouth in that given time. I'm sure that in this area many obese people could set imposing records, but if we were to set specific limits on how long we could sit at the table while eating, we would surely influence the amount of food we ate. If we were to add the element of another simultaneous activity, such as dinner conversation and perhaps a certain protocol of eating technique dictated by varying social situations, we would also influence the amount of food eaten.

Certainly our eating habits are influenced by a social situation. But I've read a myriad of scientific papers having to do with the intake of food, and I've yet to come across one entitled "A Comparative Study of Food Intake at Home Compared to That When Invited to the Boss's Home for Dinner," or "Calorie Consumption on a First Date Compared with Dates with a Steady Boyfriend." Perhaps the most interesting sociological study would be "Statistical Rates of Overeating When Visiting A Mother-in-Law."

I've never had a patient walk into my office eating an ice cream cone. Yet the people I see often label themselves "compulsive eaters." I've always equated "compulsive" with "uncontrollable." If their desire is so uncontrollable, how is it that I have never had a patient whip a fried chicken leg out of her purse and start munching on it while I was examining her? Where is the compulsion? If it were truly uncontrollable, she couldn't resist; but the truth is she resists very well. She would be too embarrassed to do otherwise!

These same "compulsive eaters" do not eat popcorn in church or hot dogs at funerals. Their compulsion is confined to convenient times when the only penalty is fat.

But with fiber in your diet, even these social situations and personal compulsions would be far less harmful than they are right now. The addition of fiber definitely prolongs the time that it takes to eat a given quantity of food. An example of this is to compare the time it takes to eat a slice of whole wheat bread to the time it takes to eat a slice of white bread. The distinction is rather subtle and not obvious unless you look for it. I tried this recently and was amazed to find how long it took to chew a slice of whole wheat bread. White bread is gone in a few chews and a few seconds. It's easy. But the whole wheat bread requires work. This same experiment was performed in England on a group of people who did not know they were the subjects of an experiment. The results were presented in a scientific paper and showed that it takes considerably longer to eat whole wheat bread than white bread.

If this principle of added fiber were expanded to include virtually all the foods you eat, it could greatly reduce the amount of high calorie food you consume. The net experience of sitting at the table for a period of time and chewing, chewing, and chewing some more succeeds in "fooling" the body into believing that it has eaten a greater quantity than it actually has. Again, my choice of words is perhaps unfortunate, for if the eating of high-fiber foods is the natural state, then it is on your present diet that your body is being fooled. Your present low-fiber diet does not give your mouth any clue as to the large number of calories passing through it, since so little effort is expended in getting refined food through your mouth and into your stomach. When you eat a naturally bulky, unprocessed food, your perception of what you have consumed will be correct, and your body will be satisfied with fewer calories.

In truth, the natural, normal diet is high in fiber and does not contain the large number of usable calories and carbohydrates you usually eat. When your ancestors consumed a diet that contained fiber, the calories and carbohydrates their bodies actually received formed only a fraction of the food that was eaten. But today almost everything you put in your mouth is digestible and absorbed by the body, and this excess consumption of calories is a major cause of our society's problem with excess fat.

If we do not change our ways, this dilemma could expand and reach a dramatic climax a century from now, when the science fiction dream of synthetic foods may be reached. Imagine that all the calories, carbohydrates, and protein you need for one meal would be packed into one super-processed, super-refined, super-compressed food capsule. This capsule would be today's processed, refined foods taken to their ultimate limit.

Imagine sitting down to dinner with your family. Resting on a small plate in front of you would be your capsule. A small, delicate spoon on a napkin next to it would be the only utensil you would need to "eat" your meal. Lifting your capsule in your spoon, you would put it on your tongue, swallow it with a gulp of water, and then finish the glass of water to quench your thirst. But you would still be hungry. "Give me another capsule," you would say. "I need to eat some more because I'm still hungry."

And you would, of course, be very hungry, for what capsule can adequately substitute for a meal? But after your second capsule you would not be less hungry, even though you had just eaten a whole second meal. A moment later your unrelieved hunger pangs would stab you again, and you would reach over, grab the bottle of pills, and pour a pile of them on your plate.

You can easily see how absurd this situation could get, and

why these pills will never be developed. The average meal would have to consist of several dozen capsules, and the calorie intake for just one meal might run as high as 30,000 or 40,000 calories! What a nation of blimps we would be!

Even though we don't have these synthetic pills to eat today, our refined and processed foods have already started us down the road to this absurd predicament. Sugar is 100 percent carbohydrate with no bulk. Our bodies are regularly "fooled" by the processed foods that monopolize our diets. We eat a sandwich on white bread. Of course we are still hungry because the white bread and the few thin slices of luncheon meat and processed cheese went down too easily. We neither had to chew it much to swallow it, nor did we feel full from eating it. Like the pills of tomorrow, the sandwich fails to convince our bodies that we have eaten as much as we have actually consumed, because our bodies instinctively demand the fibrous bulk on which our digestive systems evolved. So to get that feeling that we have eaten "enough," we eat another sandwich, or a bowl of soup, have an order of french fries on the side, and perhaps a piece of pie after the meal.

You would feel satisfied if you were to eat a meal of part fiber and part usable food. After eating the proper amount of fiber-free foods, you feel so empty that you are compelled to go on eating. Just like the science fiction drama of thirty pills for dinner, overeating by twenty-nine meals, your diet of fiber-free foods has already condemned you to a similar fate. You load your stomach with easily digestible soup, french fries, sandwiches on white bread, and pie, and you stuff yourself with calories that represent more than one meal. Then, after you have eaten double or triple your dose of calories, your food passes abnormally slowly through your digestive system. There is plenty of time to extract every last calorie out of the food, and obesity develops.

As if this weren't enough, our society prizes thinness as the appearance of health and attractiveness. But with fiber-free diets, thin bodies often come only at the price of semi-starvation. Instead of eating the normal, satisfying meal on which our bodies evolved, part fiber and part nutrients, with proper transit time and easy weight maintenance, we run schizophrenically after thinness, eating too many calories without even realizing it. No wonder obesity strikes more than half of us.

Like Alice in Wonderland, we have to "run faster and faster just to stay in the same place." And the comment I have often heard, "Doctor, I eat like a bird but I just can't seem to lose weight," should now make as much sense to you as it does to me.

It has become clear that the whole idea of supplying the American people with refined foods and then demanding that they be thin, healthy, and attractive has a serious flaw in it. We need to go back to the drawing board, to understand what has happened to our food, and try to make our eating habits work *for* us again.

Reaching for the origins of our dilemma, we can see that our food industry is part of a much larger project of commerce and industry, and that is to make life easier for us. Every year thousands of new inventions are patented, each with the object of making something easier. Manual turning of the crank on a pencil sharpener has been replaced by an electric sharpener that turns its own crank. Not only do we avoid the work of hanging clothes on a line to dry and then taking them down, but we don't even have to walk to turn off the clothes dryer, since it turns itself off.

Similarly, our food has been "manufactured" for us so that we can eat the greatest quantity with the least effort. We can eat ounces of sugar in the form of candy bars in a matter of minutes, but if we were called upon to eat the same quantity of sugar in its natural state, we would have to suffer through perhaps a pound of sugar beets. I doubt that any of us would do this, but if we did, we would be quite satisfied.

Our bread is refined so that it doesn't have to be chewed, our meat is tenderized so that it can be eaten with no work, and our corn is squashed, ground, and boiled so that we can extract from it the pure food, the pure starch that has led to the pure fat that envelops us.

It is not only the manufacturers who create the problem—we do it ourselves. What could be more natural than drinking freshly squeezed orange juice? But is it natural? Certainly I have no argument with eating an orange, but what about the orange juice? It is not the same thing. It is not only industry that refines sugar, but you do it with oranges when you squeeze them for juice. This concentrates the sweetness and extracts the calories, so that you don't have to suffer through the pulp, the fiber, and the chewing, indeed the work of pulling the orange apart. Slogans such as "Drink your orange this morning," and "The Natural Breakfast Drink" gives us a misleading impression of orange juice. And soon, when I explain my new tables, don't be surprised when you find some interesting revelations when you compare whole oranges with orange juice.

Our society seems to be moving ahead on the road to science-fiction food pills. Soon your food may be so refined, so creamy, so grain-free, so free of nondigestible bulk, and so easy to eat that you will unavoidably double and triple your daily intake of calories without even taking a single bite. Perhaps your teeth will become as useless as your appendix. Perhaps just as the surgeon routinely removes an infected appendix, you may decide to have each tooth pulled when it gets a cavity.

The consumption of sugar in this country has already risen dramatically over the years. It is presently over 105 pounds per year for each person. Since that amount is an average, it includes all kinds of people who do not eat sugar, such as those who consciously won't eat it, babies who obviously don't eat 105 pounds per year, or people in nursing homes and institutions who are on regulated diets. It is obvious, therefore, that most walking-about adults probably eat much more than 105 pounds per year. But even if we consider only 105 pounds per person, this breaks down to about two pounds per week, or over a quarter of a pound every day.

Does it really feel like you're eating four full ounces, almost a sugar-bowl full, of refined sugar every day? Of course it doesn't, but that's the danger you face. Eating that quarter of a pound in the form of cake frosting or doughnuts, in soft drinks or candy bars, gives you no impression at all of how many calories you've ingested. These sugar-filled foods provide excess calories, because you generally eat the usual amount of real food anyway. If you drink a soda with dinner instead of a glass of water, you consume the same amount of liquid but receive hundreds of extra calories. Then, after a full meal, you usually manage to find "a little extra room" for dessert.

If you were to eat your quarter of a pound of sugar-calories in the form of foods that naturally contain sugar, such as sugar beets or apples, you would see the tremendous quantity of fiber that is removed by refining. You would have to eat twenty apples, after which you certainly wouldn't feel like eating anything else. Or, you would have to eat two and a half pounds of sugar beets, and this would probably become your entire food intake for that day.

Of course, all this doesn't mean that you shouldn't eat any processed or refined foods. For one thing we must differentiate between those who are trying to lose weight and those who are trying to maintain a weight that they have already achieved. These two situations have to be handled differently.

If you're trying to lose weight, obviously you must be much more careful. What you have to remember is that you can easily correct your diet. It is not the refining and processing that is inherently bad, it is what has been refined and processed out of the foods that causes the problem. You can put this fiber back in and make your meals health restoring and weight maintaining once again.

As I've said, I am going to introduce a new food supplement that will help you to achieve this for yourself. Let's begin with wheat, because refining has done it great nutritional damage. Earlier I mentioned that a kernel of wheat can be divided into three sections. The white flour and white bread so common today are made from only one section of the wheat kernel, the endosperm. This is essentially a carbohydrate in the form of starch. It contains very little fiber. In other words, when you eat white bread, you are eating almost pure calories in a food that is constipating, and its calories are almost completely received by your body.

The bulk of the fiber contained in wheat is in the outer coating, which is called bran. This "natural bran" is not the same bran that you know as the breakfast cereal, although the breakfast product is made from it. Crude wheat bran does not resemble the processed cereal brans to which sugar is often added. In fact, crude bran is a unique substance you may have never seen before. It is light-brown colored, flaky, and flourlike. It has very little taste. If you were to put some in your mouth, you would be more impressed with the texture than the taste. It doesn't even feel like food. It does not dissolve quickly, and you might not feel like chewing it. If, however, it is properly prepared and mixed with other foods, it becomes an innocuous but valuable addition, and its slight but subtle flavor enhances the other foods with which it is cooked.

This crude wheat bran was at first the discarded portion of the wheat. Later, it was discovered to be valuable for the feeding of cattle, and still later it found its way into cereal boxes where it was improperly labeled a laxative. Bran, in fact, is only the fiber that is contained in the whole wheat kernel, and it is usually removed by refining.

Bran offers so much fiber and has so much value in a program for ending obesity and restoring health that it has become the most important food addition in this new theory of nutrition. Because of bran's unique properties as an all-around source of dietary fiber, I use it as the cornerstone of my new program. By using it and other specific foods, you can return the fiber you need to your diet.

What are the unique properties of bran? Let us look at its composition. Two cups of bran flakes weigh about 100 grams, or a little less than 4 ounces. Many calorie charts base the caloric content of foods upon 100-gram quantities. Although various authorities differ on the exact composition of bran, I shall accept the fact that it contains about 312 calories per 100 grams. Most of these calories are a result of the carbohydrate contained in the bran. Analysis shows that these 100 grams of bran contain about 53 grams of carbohydrate and 12 grams of crude fiber. We can see from this that bran is not a particularly low-calorie food.

If we compare the calories contained in apples, for example, with the calories contained in an equal weight of bran, we would find that the apples contained 58 calories, and the bran contains about five times the calories of apples. A simple calorie-counting approach would suggest that apples are a much better diet food than bran; it would actually suggest that apples are five times as good.

However, let's look at the other ingredient we've been discussing, fiber. Note these comparisons.

BRAN COMPARED TO APPLES

Per 100 Gms	Calories	Carbohydrate (gms)	Fiber (gms)
Bran	312	53	12
Apples (1 small, 2 inches in diameter)	54	14	1

There is twelve times as much fiber in the bran as there is in the apples.

Which is the better diet food? Is there anyone who will dispute that apples are a good diet food? I doubt it. It's universally accepted as such, although there are a small number of diet books that disparage apples. Bran is also a good diet food, even though it contains several times the calories of apples, because bran supplies something in quantity that the apples do not—fiber. As I have pointed out, it is this fiber that will act as an appetite depressant by its sheer bulk, and by the work and time required to eat it. It is this fiber that is going to speed up the journey of all your food through your intestinal tract, so that your body receives fewer calories. And it is this fiber that will tie up and carry out of your system potentially toxic substances caused by bacterial decomposition, which may someday loom large as the thieves of your life.

The question, "Which is better?" must be answered, "Neither." Each possesses a quality that is indispensable. Before you opened this book you were well aware that you could not eat unlimited calories and expect to lose weight. Apples, by substituting for higher calorie foods, help you decrease your caloric intake. But you also knew that by eating a low-calorie diet, you simply weren't eating enough food. You were still hungry. You paid the price of extra calories when you tried to stop your hunger pangs by taking extra bites of food and ingesting extra calories.

Just imagine for a moment what you would wish for as a perfect solution to your diet-hunger problems. You would want a substance that added bulk to your meals and let you eat more without gaining weight. You would want it to be easy to add to your meals, almost a nonfood that still tasted good. You would want it to give you the feeling that you had eaten a "solid meal" when it was inside you, being digested. And as a bonus, you would want it to make a contribution to good health, perhaps helping prevent some of the serious diseases to which refined foods contribute. High-fiber bran answers this wish perfectly.

The reason why bran answers this wish is amazing. It may even reinforce your gloom about the way our society works. We industrially removed fiber from our foods to improve it. We raised several generations on this new, refined-food diet. And we discovered ourselves confronting immense problems in obesity and disease epidemics that now appear to be directly related to our eating habits. We also discovered that nature contains a miracle substance that might rid our society of most obesity problems and eliminate what seems to be the causes of many dread diseases. What does this miracle substance turn out to be? Lo and behold! The miracle substance is the very same fiber that we removed from food in the first place!

The natural world will always remain one step ahead of our industrial ingenuity. Our bodies are part of this natural world. They evolved in it and they stay healthier when we remain part of it. I will forever be awed by how much better our bodies and the world work when we are not recklessly tampering with them.

Unfortunately there is no way for the eating habits for Americans living in our super-technological society to "return to nature" overnight. You are forced to walk in the back door, through a "high-fiber diet" that returns to your body the dietary fiber manufacturers have taken out.

This book has a twin purpose. Most important and immediate, it explains how you can easily and quickly return a sufficient amount of fiber to your diet.

But the book also introduces a greater, more rewarding purpose. In Chapter 9, I offer a plan for encouraging the food industry—manufacturers, restauranteurs, etc.—to join with nutritionally concerned Americans in making our foods the part-fiber, part-nutrient bundles they should be. Hopefully, this will be a widespread and successful program that will help millions of Americans return fiber to their meals.

The first part of this two-pronged effort is like a bandage covering a wound. With a minimum of effort, each of you can add adequate amounts of fiber to your own diet. Then together we can go on to the second step: healing the wound. We might be able to cause enough manufactured products to change, and change some of the offerings of restaurants so that the fiber we need will be available to everyone who wants it. Admittedly, this second program has a long-range goal. But it is an effort we cannot avoid if we hope to rid our society of many of its obesity problems and attain substantially improved health.

Certainly by now you suspect that your diet requires more than a smidgen of fiber. In fact, you probably suspect—and rightly so—that there is a minimum amount of fiber that you should take in with each and every meal. Later I will suggest many good-tasting ways to do this and a variety of foods that provide fiber. But for now, I will explain the easiest way to begin this dietary change.

I just spoke of bran and its unique properties. Soon I will explain how you can add bran to your meals and eat greater quantities of food than on other diets, yet still lose weight. For this natural program of weight loss, bran is as close to being a "perfect food for dieters" (and weight maintainers) as nature offers. For Americans used to eating refined-food diets, it is as perfect a source of easily usable dietary fiber as anyone could hope to find. I will show you just how good it is in a minute.

But first, I have to admit that we have not reached perfection. As a result, you must learn how to evaluate all foods and see their fibrous value as well as their limits. Bran will certainly not be the only source of fiber in your diet. So that you will be able to do this evaluation for yourself, in the tables in Chapter 12 you will find a new concept I have invented—a new number—that clarifies the amount of fiber in food and shows the food's usefulness as a diet food.

This number relates the fiber content of food to its carbohydrate content. In order to make your job easier, and to eliminate the need for an electronic calculator next to your knife and fork, I have computed this new number for you. It is called the carbohydrate-fiber ratio. Its abbreviation is C/F.

The C/F is a comparison of the number of grams of available carbohydrate of a food to the number of grams of fiber it contains. It is arrived at by dividing the available carbohydrate by the fiber. The resulting number tells us how good for dieting and weight maintenance each food really is.

Most people have dieted at one time or another. For those who tried to consume fewer calories or simply tried to eat less food, this ratio fits right in with their attitudes. The lower the C/F, the better the food is for dieting, because the higher it is in fiber. Unlike the fast weight-loss diets you are used to, however, the more foods you select with low carbohydrate-fiber ratios, the more food you can eat.

In the case of bran, the carbohydrate-fiber ratio is calculated by dividing 53 grams by 12 grams.

THE C/F OF BRAN

$$C/F\ (Bran) = \frac{Grams\ of\ Carbohydrate\ in\ Bran}{Grams\ of\ Fiber\ in\ Bran} = {}^{53}\!/_{12} = 4.4$$

The result, 4.4, is, in general, a very good, low C/F.

If this sends you running for your high school math book, don't go. It isn't necessary. Refer to the tables in Chapter 12. There you will find not only the calorie content of foods but also the carbohydrate content, the fiber content, and most important, the carbohydrate-fiber ratio.

Let us calculate the C/F for apples.

THE C/F OF APPLES

$$C/F\ (Apples) = \frac{Grams\ of\ Carbohydrate\ in\ Apples}{Grams\ of\ Fiber\ in\ Apples} = {}^{14}\!/_{1} = 14$$

You can see from this that the C/F for apples is 14, which is about three times as high as that of bran. What does this tell you about the two foods? It tells you that bran is proportionately more fibrous than apples; that the calories in bran are not as naked as the calories in apples. In general, you should give preference in your diet to bran when there is a choice between it and apples. It is unlikely, however, that you would ever have to make a choice between these two foods. I have used them only as examples.

Does this tell you that apples are not a good diet food? No, not at all. It simply tells you that bran is better in some ways.

In fact, to see this ratio and know what it means is to learn something revolutionary. The C/F is a real breakthrough in understanding what good nutrition really should be for all of us. The new numbers in Chapter 12, the carbohydrate-fiber ratios, make good dieting and good health more attainable than ever before. They make it possible to eat meals containing more good-tasting, enjoyable food than you ever dreamed you would be allowed. They help you lose weight at a reasonably fast rate by directing you to the specific foods that contain the most fiber.

If this isn't the biggest nutritional and dieting breakthrough that's come along while I've been a doctor, I'll eat my book—which by the way isn't a bad idea, since these pages contain a lot of indigestible vegetable fiber. But I won't have to do this, because this breakthrough *is* the biggest and the most important. It combines all that dieters and nutritionists have searched in vain for: solid meals, good food, sound nutrition, the chance for greatly improved health, easy weight maintenance, and the biggest bonus of all, easy weight loss. And I am certain that medical authorities will agree: this is one diet that cannot be criticized as being nutritionally deficient.

In the tables in Chapter 12, there is a comparison between most of the foods that you commonly eat. Keep in mind that this comparison applies only to foods that are of plant origin. Foods of animal origin contain none of this fiber, and therefore cannot be considered under these same rules. They will be discussed separately.

Let us look at the following table comparing foods of greatly varying fiber content. The ten foods it considers will also be found in the tables in Chapter 12.

Let us examine the column marked fiber. You will note immediately that bran stands alone in fiber content among this group of foods. That is why it is mentioned so extensively and

SAMPLE TABLE

Food (Per 100 gms)	C/F	Fiber (gms)	Carbohydrate (gms)	Calories
Avocados	2.9	1.6	4.7	161
Bread (white)	254.0	0.2	50.0	267
Bran	4.4	12.0	53.0	312
Mushrooms	4.5	0.8	3.6	25
Oranges	24.0	0.5	12.0	47
Orange Juice (fresh)	100.0	0.1	10.0	45
Peanuts	11.0	1.5	17.0	560
Potatoes	34.0	0.5	17.0	76
Raisins	76.0	1.0	76.0	286
Raspberries	3.7	3.0	11.0	45

used so prominently in the recipes in this book. All factors considered, it is nature's single best source of fiber.

Look at the calorie column. Note the vast difference in the calorie content of mushrooms and peanuts. Before you resolve never to eat another peanut, consider this. I shall allow you to eat peanuts as part of your program for maintaining normal weight, but they cannot be eaten on The High-Fiber Reducing Diet. You will note that peanuts are somewhat higher than mushrooms in the C/F column. But peanuts also have many more calories. That is why they are only allowed on The Weight-Maintenance Diet, while mushrooms are also recommended on the weight-loss diet.

Now let us look at another interesting revelation brought out by these comparisons. What are the relative merits of oranges and orange juice? Oranges have a C/F of 24, which is rather high when compared with mushrooms. But now look at orange juice. It has a C/F of 100. Why is there such a difference? The answer lies in the processing. In the case of orange juice, processing consists of squeezing the orange. The result? You've squeezed out the sugar and left behind most of the fiber.

How does orange juice work to your disadvantage, from a practical standpoint? The figures for oranges in the table represent one orange. For orange juice the figures represent a little over three ounces, not even half a cup. It is the juice of more than one squeezed orange. What does it take to ingest that tiny quantity of orange juice? Probably one or two swallows. Look how easily the orange juice goes down. You drink it as a prelude to breakfast or as a beverage. In no way does it substitute for the breakfast. It is simply a high-calorie addition. A few swallows and all the calories contained in two or three oranges are down the hatch and now you can get ready for the serious business of eating breakfast.

There's a big difference when you eat a whole orange. Do you think you will be able to dispose of it with one or two swallows? Hardly. Not only must you peel it, but you have to cut it in sections or perhaps pull it apart. You'll do a lot of chewing, with the result that several minutes will pass before you have finished with that orange. When you are done you will be required to dispose of the skin, seeds, and some pulp, which is another task in itself. Instead of drinking a glass of orange juice with your breakfast, had you eaten those two or three oranges directly, they probably would have constituted your entire breakfast.

The sum total of comparing these two activities, that is, eating the orange and drinking its juice, is obvious. Drinking the orange juice will not inform your body of the calories it has just ingested. Indeed, it will delude you into thinking that you haven't done much more than consume a glass of flavored water. Eating two or three oranges will give your body its truthful perspective. You have eaten a certain amount of high-energy food and you've put forth the effort to prove it. Drinking a glass of orange juice probably encouraged drinking another and another. In fact, you are probably drinking too much of this potent liquid on a regular basis. Eating oranges is better for your weight, because you are receiving a smaller amount of calories and a higher amount of fiber. Your digestive system also feels more comfortable with the fiber and pulp you have eaten than it does with the potent, high-calorie glass of orange juice.

I could go on with such examples, but the real value is in showing you how easy it is to decide what to eat and what not to eat. Just look at the C/F for these two foods. For oranges it is 24, for orange juice it is 100. This tells the whole story in an instant. It places oranges well within the range of acceptable foods. It places orange juice just on the fringe of unacceptability.

What are the limits of acceptability? At this point I am only going to give you a general idea. For The High-Fiber Reducing Diet, the upper limit of acceptability is 25. For The Weight-Maintenance Diet, the upper limit is 100. However, there is more to these diets than just watching these two numbers, as you will presently see. For the vast majority of readers my standards will prove accurate. For some, these standards will have to be altered and tailored to the individual.

You will use these standards according to what you are trying to accomplish. If you are trying to lose weight, you will be looking at lower C/F values. If you are trying to maintain your proper weight and enjoy general good health, you will be allowed higher C/F foods. There will also be some foods that are never permitted.

What about bread? The table shows white enriched bread. (Other breads are covered in Chapter 12.) In the C/F department white bread wins the booby prize. Why? Because the fiber it contains is negligible, and the carbohydrates are formidable. You can inhale its 267 calories with little more effort than drinking orange juice. Because of the absence of fiber, it is going to drag its way through your body at a snail's pace. You'll probably absorb every last one of those calories, and you'll probably feel as though you haven't eaten a thing.

I can no more allow you to eat this poison than I can allow you to drink cyanide. But before you go into mourning, remember that white bread is not the only kind of bread. Later

I'm going to speak of others that are more acceptable, and give first prize to whole wheat bread—that is, bread that still contains almost all of its fiber.

Now, some final observations on this table. You can see why raisins, in spite of all that iron, aren't that healthy a food. Their C/F ratio is 76. How about raspberries? Does that surprise you? They have one of the lowest C/F values, and they are relatively low in calories. In case you've been peering lustily at avocados with that C/F of 2.9, let me stop you before you run out and buy a truck load to begin your diet. Avocados are permitted on The Weight-Maintenance Diet, but not on the reducing diet, because there are too many calories derived from fat in avocados.

Let us move on to the basic principle involved in losing and maintaining proper weight. On The High-Fiber Reducing Diet, losing weight is accomplished by eating an adequate amount of fiber daily and keeping the calorie intake at a reasonable level. You burn up a smaller amount of calories per day, but, because of the breakthrough of a high-fiber diet, you can eat a greater quantity of food than is generally recommended by authorities for weight loss.

My theory is that weight loss will be accomplished automatically if you take in sufficient fiber daily, if you eat virtually no refined carbohydrates or refined sugar in any form, and if you eliminate unusually high-calorie foods from your meals. You can then eat larger quantities of foods that contain a large percentage of fiber and are low in calories. You will not have to rigidly count calories because, with sufficient bulk in your meals, your food will pass through you quickly and your body will automatically limit the number of calories it receives.

The Weight-Maintenance Diet is similar, but with one exception. Here it is only necessary to "receive" as many calories as you burn up. Since you will be following the same general rule just mentioned for weight loss—eating an adequate amount of fiber daily—the main practical difference is you will have access to a wide variety of foods.

You will soon see that with fiber in your meals, the whole

concept of what is a diet food and what is not will expand enormously—to your benefit and pleasure. High fiber is the key to a whole new world of better eating, while controlling your weight at the same time.

Now let's see how you will enter this healthier world on a day-to-day basis.

CHAPTER 6

HOW YOU WILL INTRODUCE FIBER INTO YOUR DIET

The need to add fiber to your diet is a new discovery, developed from observation of primitive societies in which a diet high in fiber is widely accepted. I have "Americanized" this diet by providing you a variety of quick and easy ways to get your necessary fiber.

Why is this Americanization necessary? Years of observation of thousands of obese patients have taught me which dietary adjustments are realistic and which are not. Most people simply wouldn't listen if I asked them to return to the laboriously prepared meals of their great-great-grandparents. Their leisure time, their jobs, and their varied activities have become too valuable. No amount of health and weight benefits will get millions of people to again cage themselves in a hot kitchen endlessly baking loaves of high-fiber bread, canning their own carefully selected vegetables, and nutritionally planning each and every meal.

Also, Americans like the kinds of convenience foods they presently eat or they wouldn't be eating them. The food companies have not persuaded us—we have chosen to eat the foods that please us most.

If you are to get the fiber you need, it must be Americanized and made into a supplement to be added to the kinds of meals you currently eat. By patient planning, combined with my knowledge of what is needed, this has been accomplished successfully. You will see how you can get the thinner appearance and increased health you seek with almost no sacrifice at all. In fact, you may save some money in your family's food budget.

How much fiber should you eat? We know, for example, that the African Zulus who provided us with some valuable data ate as much as 25 grams of fiber a day. This is a considerable amount. We would have to eat almost nothing but fibrous foods to equal it. It is not likely that Americans will eat this kind of diet, no matter who recommends it. It is not even advisable for anyone to attempt to, unless they gradually accustom themselves to large amounts of fiber and approach this nearly total fiber diet very slowly.

Most Americans are used to eating only small amounts of fiber. I will therefore recommend that their diet include as much fiber as possible. I believe that those Americans who eat what they feel is a maximum amount of fiber will not even reach the minimum amount eaten by the rural Zulus. Yet for our society, the maxim can safely be, "the more the better."

I will set an American minimum of 10 to 12 grams of fiber a day. Since the average American already consumes 3 to 5 grams of fiber daily, this means an addition of only 7 grams of fiber a day.

This 7 extra grams is a magic number. It is only one third of the difference between our fiber consumption and that of the rural African's. (There is a 20- to 22-gram difference.) Yet when you add 7 grams to your present 3- to 5-gram intake, you just about equal half the 25-gram fiber intake of the rural Zulu. For most of us, these 10 to 12 grams of fiber will prove adequate for weight maintenance and health protection. For losing weight, we combine this fiber with a reduced caloric intake.

Because our digestive systems are not accustomed to even this amount of fiber, you can best adjust to 7 extra grams a day during a gradual, two-week build-up. The overenthusiastic reader who attempts to shorten this time runs the risk of discomfort and abandoning fiber before he has given it a fair chance. So don't be too gung ho when you can reach both weight maintenance and health sensibly and comfortably.

The easiest way to add this extra fiber to your diet is through a high-fiber supplement to the foods you already eat. Since you are probably already preparing the kind of dishes that I recommend, there will be very few new cooking skills to learn. You will only have to reach for a jar or bag of fiber supplement —natural, unprocessed bran flakes—and scoop the suggested number of heaping tablespoons into the foods you cook.

In the next chapter and in the recipes in Chapter 11 I will show you many delicious ways to add fiber to your meals. In many dishes you won't even know it is there! But for the immediate transition period, there is an easier way to get your fiber. This is to eat it in the form of bran in a soup or broth just before your meals.

By the way (and this is a point I will stress later when I get to the reducing and the weight-maintenance diets) you should see your doctor before embarking on this or any other weight-loss program. It is impossible for me to know your exact physical condition or your personal medical history, but these factors should be taken into consideration whenever you begin a diet of any kind. See your doctor. Let him or her advise you before you begin.

If the extra 7 grams of fiber come exclusively from wheat bran, then it is necessary to eat 2.14 ounces (60 grams) of bran flakes a day. This equals nine heaping tablespoons of bran flakes per day, or, if finely ground bran is used, only six heaping tablespoons.

The difference between coarse bran and fine bran is simple but important. Coarse bran is what you buy at the health-food store. It is acceptable for all the dishes in the recipe section, but fine bran is somewhat easier to use.

Fine bran is made by grinding coarse bran in an electric grinder. I know of four brands of grinders on the market, ranging in price from about $12 to about $20. There are two advantages to using fine bran. First, it is ground into a rather fine powder so it is more concentrated and you use fewer tablespoons to get the same amount. Second, since the particles are smaller, in many dishes it becomes totally imperceptible.

After the two-week gradual initiation period, you should develop the habit of having your fiber in the form of nine heaping tablespoons of bran every day (or six tablespoons of fine bran). This should be distributed among the three meals, so three heaping tablespoons should be added to each meal.

The daily use of this diet will teach you which foods are high in fiber and which have very little fiber. Then, you can use other high-fiber foods to substitute for part of your bran. But to start, consider all other fibrous foods as "extra fiber" and three heaping tablespoons of bran at each meal as your minimum requirement. This way, you will always be sure of getting enough fiber, and you will not have to push yourself to learn quickly how to count grams of fiber. By using bran as a supplement in each meal, you will get all the fiber supplement you need. You don't even have to learn to count grams of fiber as long as you keep using bran instead.

I have just mentioned adding bran to a soup or broth that is taken before each meal. I particularly like this way of eating bran because it acts as an appetite depressant. This high-fiber soup can be made very easily, with a minimum of effort. There are various broth products on the market, such as bouillon cubes or broth powders, and they come in several flavors. They are usually prepared instantly by adding a bouillon cube or a teaspoon of powder to a cup of boiling water. This produces a flavorful, low-calorie cup of soup. Three heaping tablespoons of bran are added to this. You now have an even more flavorful and considerably thicker soup.

If there is any objection to it, it will probably be the texture. After a lifetime of eating super-smooth refined foods, you may not instantly adapt to the coarser texture of fibrous foods. You are used to hearing about "tender" steaks, the "smoothest" peanut butter, and the "creamiest" pudding. Potato chips may contain preservatives to keep them "crunchy," but once you have started to chew them they are processed to break down into a soft goo like other foods.

Fibrous foods are different, there is no question about that. Their texture reflects their component parts, the tougher cell walls that are processed out of the refined foods you are used to eating. When you chew these coarser foods, think about an older and wiser period in human nutrition, the eons that preceded the last century, before machines removed the fiber that you are seriously chewing again for the first time.

You can begin to experience this for yourself by making a cup of broth and adding one heaping teaspoon of bran, the quantity of fiber you will consume before each meal for the first three days.

I think you will find the soup more flavorful, thicker, and tastier than the broth alone. Most important, this gives you an immediate way of getting the minimum requirement of fiber into your diet with a minimum of effort. This soup can be eaten with each meal, even breakfast, although you probably will prefer to incorporate the bran into your breakfast in ways more consistent with traditional American breakfasts.

Once you taste this soup or other foods to which fiber has been added, you will probably find that eating foods with texture is not at all objectionable. In fact, it will soon start to feel natural.

If you do find the texture of the bran-bouillon mixture objectionable, it can be improved by boiling for ten or fifteen minutes. This softens the bran and makes its texture similar to the soft foods you are used to eating. But once you eat it regularly, you will see how easy it is to like and enjoy fiber, a familiar part of a healthier, more natural meal.

Those people willing to exert a little more effort can produce a product they may find even more appealing. This is something I find absolutely delicious. It is a mixture of bran with cooked buckwheat groats.

Buckwheat groats are a nutritious cereal product that have

been used, for the most part, as an ethnic food. Traditionally Jewish people eat large amounts of buckwheat groats, which they call kasha. It is often used as a vegetable with meals, like rice or potatoes, with gravy over it. Or it may be used as a stuffing in various types of dough, or in soups, where it adds a very rich flavor. The buckwheat groats are brown and have a rather pleasant aroma when cooked. Buckwheat is also ground into flour and is used to make buckwheat pancakes, something which I always associate with a hearty farm breakfast.

Here we have a terribly neglected product. Not only do buckwheat groats have great nutritive value, containing half the protein of meat, but they are also a delightful adjunct to a meal. As you saw in our discussion of the carbohydrate-fiber ratio, we do not lose sight of the nutrition offered by the fibrous foods we eat. Buckwheat groats have a protein content that may prove very important in our inflation-ridden society.

Both bran and buckwheat groats are relatively inexpensive. In addition, they add bulk to the meal. Consuming them in a broth or mixed in the meal substitutes for part of the more expensive plant foods and even some of the meat that you would otherwise consume. High-fiber meals produce the feeling of being "full," of having eaten a "solid meal," a feeling that fiber helps you obtain at a lower cost than with high-calorie, processed foods.

As I said before, an added nutritional benefit comes from the protein content of buckwheat groats. Other fibrous foods also contain significant amounts of protein. Whole wheat bread contains more protein than white bread.

When you add a fiber supplement to your food you accomplish several goals at once. You can reduce the intake of other more expensive plant foods. Second, you can reduce somewhat the quantity of meat you eat because buckwheat groats add protein to the meal. You have probably been cautioned repeatedly against eating excessive amounts of red meats because of their high caloric content, about 100 calories per ounce. Using fiber is an inexpensive way to cut down on the quantity of these meats but still get sufficient protein in your diet. Buckwheat groats and whole wheat bread are just two of many ways to do this.

To those readers whose incomes are fairly high, the cost of various foods may not seem important. But in many families, even many middle-class families, parents must feed themselves and their children with "filling" foods—bread, inexpensive pastries, and reduced portions of meat—because their income no longer supports the kind of eating they enjoyed in preinflationary years.

From an economic standpoint, one important benefit from adding fibrous bran and buckwheat groats to your meals is that you will be eating better for less money. In families on very tight budgets, where "eat less" has become an unavoidable necessity, dietary fiber can provide added bulk to meals and nutritionally help supplement deficient diets. In the original findings that brought out this new information, the rural Zulus ate 90 percent fibrous foods, yet were healthier in many ways than the urban Zulus. This is not being patronizing. When your family doesn't have the money to eat all it wants, a carefully planned supplement of inexpensive fibrous foods can make a vital contribution to improving the nutritional quality of the diet, while giving you and your children the satisfaction of eating regular, solid meals.

If you are somewhat better off financially, these food savings can be used in other ways. You may want to substitute an occasional steak for hamburger. Or you may have asparagus one night instead of peas. Or you may use your savings to serve a juicy, fresh melon for dessert.

Adding fiber to your meals will certainly not reverse the effects of inflation, but it will give hard-pressed families a new way to hold down the all-too-explosive food budget while improving their family's weight maintenance and health at the same time. And it will give many middle-class families a new way to save a little money, or perhaps eat a little better.

When I first became interested in adding fiber to my diet, it was a delightful surprise to find that the flavor of buckwheat groats blends very well with wheat bran. The resulting mixture retains the original flavor of the buckwheat groats. Together they offer excellent nutrition, high fiber, and a multitude of cooking possibilities.

An optimum mixture of the two to achieve high-fiber content is accomplished by mixing three parts of bran to one part of buckwheat groats, by volume. (Buy a small box of buckwheat groats to make sure you like them. Bran picks up the flavor of whatever food it is in, but buckwheat groats have a distinctive flavor of their own.) When cooked, the resulting mixture looks, tastes, and smells exactly like the buckwheat groats but has the added advantage of being extremely high in dietary fiber.

This mixture can be substituted for bran alone and added to broth. You must use seven heaping tablespoons of the cooked mixture to supply your minimum 2.3 grams of fiber to that meal.

For people who find it tasty, the buckwheat-bran mixture can become a staple for this new way of eating. If sweetened with artificial sweetener, it makes a delicious hot or cold breakfast cereal. It can be used as a vegetable with lunch or dinner, makes an excellent stuffing for fowl when prepared with cooked, chopped vegetables (onions, carrots, celery, mushrooms, etc.), and can be mixed with ground beef, chopped chicken, fish, cheese, or a variety of vegetables to produce tantalizing casseroles.

I would recommend that each household keep a large jar of this basic food in the refrigerator and replenish it frequently. In Chapter 11 there are detailed instructions on how to prepare and store this mixture.

Bran and the bran-and-buckwheat mixture are the quickest, easiest, and least expensive ways of adding fiber to your diet, but they are by no means the only ways. Many other foods contain high amounts of fiber. There is coconut, for example. There are also chickpeas (garbanzo beans), sesame seeds, soy beans, parsley, watercress, and celery.

A multitude of foods are high in fiber, but their value is relative. Some also contain an amount of calories that would make them undesirable if eaten in unlimited quantities. I want you to learn to evaluate your choice of fibrous foods by means of the carbohydrate-fiber ratio. Your guiding rule is simple and clear: try to eat as much fiber as possible, but try to obtain it from the foods with the lowest carbohydrate-fiber ratios. For example, suppose your main concern is losing weight. You want to decide between two foods for breakfast, oatmeal and shredded wheat. Look at the C/F tables in Chapter 12. You will see that oatmeal has a C/F of 45 and shredded wheat, 35. Just because both foods are permissible does not mean they are equally good. Remember, choose the food with the lowest carbohydrate-fiber ratio. If you want a food that has a higher C/F, I will tell you how to modify it to reduce its C/F and make it just as good as a food with a lower C/F (see pp. 137–138). But unless you modify the food with the higher C/F, eat the one with the lower C/F.

If you ingest 7 extra grams of fiber each day and follow the C/F ratios, you will gain the control over your weight you have always wanted. An extra 7 grams of fiber will be enough for you although it is a minimum. I might encourage you to use more than that if you tolerate it well. It is unlikely that any significant number of Americans will reach the 25-gram-per-day fiber intake of the rural Zulu. To do this you would have to ingest three to four cups of wheat bran daily or its equivalent. I can't recommend this. If you were to eat that quantity of bran, I doubt that you could eat anything else. The bulk would be tremendous.

Even the bulk represented by 7 extra grams of fiber per day is considerable, and it will have a profound effect on limiting your intake of higher calorie foods. Bran swells when it absorbs water; this is why I recommend that you take it in a broth before meals, and why I will soon recommend that you drink an eight-ounce glass of water or another beverage after your meal.

As you become used to eating high-fiber meals, you will realize that bran takes up part of the available volume of your stomach, a part that was formerly occupied by the naked calories of refined foods. You will soon learn to reduce the quantity of each kind of food that you eat to compensate for the space taken by the bran. The amount of refined food you eat and the amount of calories your body receives will be regulated automatically, and you will have no need to count calories or exercise willpower.

This is a major step forward for everyone who wants to lose weight, as well as for those who find it difficult to keep their weight at its proper level. It is very hard to lose weight when you eat only refined and processed foods. To feel full on a meal of refined foods, you have to eat too many calories. Furthermore, virtually all of the naked calories find their way into your bloodstream, where they contribute to making you fat. The fibrous bulk your body expects to find when it eats a low-fiber meal is back at the factory, where it was removed in processing. Inevitably, you grow fat, a variety of diseases continue to incubate in your body, and your health declines.

When you add fiber to your meals, you add bulk and force the proportion of refined, high-C/F foods back to a normal level. A meal that includes part fiber and part nutrients is the normal diet, and it gives you the feeling that you've eaten a good, solid meal. Fibrous foods move through your body with a normal transit time. Their bulk automatically regulates your calorie and carbohydrate intake. By going back to a normal high-fiber diet you eliminate the need for rigorous calorie counting, because you are eliminating the excess calories. As a result, you wisely avoid a depressing battle between your willpower and your stomach.

I have mentioned that you will not begin taking in the extra 7 grams of fiber on your first day. You must take two weeks to reach this amount. For the first three days you should ingest one heaping teaspoon of bran flakes with each meal. On the fourth day increase this to two heaping teaspoons three times a day. On the seventh day begin using one heaping tablespoon three times a day. On the tenth day go up to two heaping tablespoons three times a day. And after two weeks increase this to three heaping tablespoonsful three times a day.

An easy way to schedule this adjustment is to mark your kitchen calendar, copying the pattern illustrated in the following chart. In the chart, Sunday is the first day you begin taking bran.

Sun.	Mon.	Tues.	Wed.	Thurs.	Fri.	Sat.
(day 1) 1 tsp.	1 tsp.	1 tsp.	2 tsp.	2 tsp.	2 tsp.	1 tbsp.
1 tbsp.	1 tbsp.	2 tbsp.	2 tbsp.	2 tbsp.	3 tbsp.	3 tbsp.

Now a word about the effect on your bowel movements. Bran has the reputation of being a laxative, and therefore you might expect to see changes in your bowel movements. I maintain that it is not a laxative, but that the effect of eating fiber, whether as bran or in other foods, is to produce the normally rapid digestive state instead of the "clockwork constipation" produced by a low-fiber diet.

You might see an increase in your number of bowel movements per day. This is not undesirable. You will undoubtedly see a difference in the size of your stools. They will be larger, lighter, and a little softer. Some patients on this diet report an excess amount of gas, but this seems to be only in the beginning phase and rarely continues beyond two or three weeks.

If any of this seems undesirable to you, consider the alternatives—obesity, cancer of the colon, heart disease, diverticulitis, polyps of the colon, peptic ulcer, diabetes, and more.

I am not joking. In your anxieties over obesity you have learned a great deal about its harmful consequences. High-blood pressure is only part of the price often paid by those who carry excess weight. We all know that high blood pressure is the "hidden killer," a main indicator of potential stroke. Obesity also causes many other health problems, but we must not overlook its emotional consequences, including loss of self-esteem, a sense of failure in defeating it, and in some patients, depression.

Even more than obesity, refined foods must bear a large share of the blame for many of the diseases that make up the Naked Calorie Disease. The rates of certain diseases in urban societies that eat a modern, super-refined diet is much higher than in those groups that eat sufficient quantities of unrefined, high-fiber foods.

You have seen that the diet of Americans has changed drastically in the last century. The use of refined sugar has risen far beyond its previous level. The consumption of bread and other grain foods has fallen, and the white bread you eat has been stripped of its fiber by refining. On top of all this, there has been a substantial decline in the consumption of fresh fruits and vegetables, which provide some fiber, and an increase in the drinking of fruit juices and eating defibered processed foods.

Consider the benefits of adding fiber and ending the monopoly of these refined foods over your meals—reduced weight, easy maintenance of your proper weight, a thinner and more attractive appearance, reduced risk of many serious diseases, greater health and well-being, a sense of self-assurance, the good after-eating feeling of a solid, natural meal, and the potential for a longer and much healthier life.

What is the key to all this? Add a minimum of 7 grams of fiber to your diet daily. You can do this most effectively by adding three heaping tablespoons of bran to each meal. Don't forget to approach this quantity gradually, over a period of two weeks.

In the next chapter and in the recipe section you will find many good-tasting ways to incorporate fiber into your meals. They are easy to try and easy to use. They'll quickly teach you how to use fiber as a dietary supplement. Be inventive and you will discover many more ways than I have suggested. I will be grateful if you will write to me to share the results of your experiences and your own culinary imagination. (My address is given in Chapter 9.) Hopefully, soon more and more Americans will be enjoying delicious meals that are once again nutritionally sound.

CHAPTER 7

THE WEIGHT-MAINTENANCE AND HEALTH-PRESERVATION DIET

Since the maintenance of your proper weight is the best contribution you can make to living a long and healthy life, it will be treated first. In Chapter 8 I will present the weight-reducing diet and tell you how to lose your excess pounds.

When you add fiber to your diet, weight maintenance accomplishes more than keeping you from getting fat. It is actually a health-preservation program that, in addition to protecting you from the disastrous results of obesity, appears to prevent the multitude of diseases that are related to our society's super-refined foods.

The weight-maintenance program given here is the basic program of this book. The weight-loss program in the next chapter is simply a variation on this weight-maintenance program. Weight is lost by creating an artificial situation for a definite, but hopefully not a prolonged period of time. It is a temporary activity that eliminates obesity, after which the more important task of weight control begins.

My real goal is much larger than the temporary elimination of obesity. It is controlling your weight and helping to permanently defeat the Naked Calorie Epidemic. In the same way that the government builds a dam to protect a river valley that loses hundreds of millions of dollars in property damage every spring when it is flooded by melting snow, our society needs to control the surging flood of diseases caused by our bad eating habits.

For you to accomplish this requires that you adopt two goals. The first is controlling your weight, and the second is preserving the health of your digestive system, and therefore of your body. When you add fiber to your diet and follow my other recommendations, you accomplish both of these goals together. But since this program is aimed at permanently ending your obesity, I have named it The Weight-Maintenance Diet.

How do you successfully accomplish this program? There are seven steps to The Weight-Maintenance Diet. I have reduced these procedures to this easy-to-follow list:

1. Eat sufficient fiber in your diet daily.
2. Distribute the fiber so you eat some with each of your three meals.
3. Do not eat refined sugar or refined flour. Use whole wheat flour or products made from whole wheat flour rather than refined flour.
4. Use artificial sweeteners when you desire sugar; if you do not use artificial sweeteners, you may substitute a small amount of honey.
5. Be sure your diet contains adequate vitamins.
6. Drink adequate fluids.
7. Get sufficient exercise.

As you can see, this is a common-sense program consistent with medically accepted, proper diet. Its difference from most diets is that it includes what scientists have recently learned about fiber and refined foods. You should have no difficulty following it if you are now eating conventionally, since it involves no extraordinary changes in meal planning.

EAT SUFFICIENT FIBER DAILY

In the last chapter I suggested that in order to enjoy the benefits of weight control and protection from certain diseases, you should add a minimum of 7 grams of fiber to your food every day. Accept this as a cardinal rule, and do not deviate. But remember, do not add all the fiber at once. Increase the use of bran gradually over a two-week period, as described in Chapter 6.

It is impossible to fix the amount of fiber that you should take in daily to adequately satisfy every individual need. In this regard, I should differentiate between the words "normal" and "average" as they are used in medicine. When the government tells you that the Recommended Daily Allowance (RDA) for Vitamin A is 5,000 IU (International Units), it is not saying that this is the amount that normal people need. It is not saying that unless your body requires exactly 5,000 IU daily you are some kind of a freak. What it is saying is that if a large group of people were tested for their requirements, the average need within this group would be 5,000 IU; some might only need 4,000 IU and others might need more than 5,000.

Likewise with fiber there may be even wider variation in individual needs. My recommendations of quantity of bran to be added to your daily diet will therefore be adequate for some and too high or too low for others.

How will you know if the amount is right for you? Your bowel habits will provide the best clue. You should have at least one bowel movement a day. More than this might be acceptable to some people. The stool, like that of the African natives studied, should be quite large, but rather soft and unformed. A more accurate criterion is transit time. Ideally, a transit time of twenty-four-to-thirty-six hours should be the goal. But how do you measure your own transit time? To accurately do this without laboratory facilities is difficult.

For those who desire to arrive at the exact amount of bran they require, I have included a simplified do-it-yourself transit time test in Appendix B. Since it is a home test it is not guaranteed accurate, but its limitations are fully discussed in the Appendix.

What do you do if you have reason to believe that you are getting too little or too much bran? Obviously you make a change. You may add or delete from your daily ration to suit your needs. The appearance of the stool and the transit time will point the way.

In Chapter 11 you will find a variety of recipes that will teach you the actual mechanics of putting bran into your food. You can use these recipes as a guide to adding bran to your own recipes.

I encountered a problem in trying to determine the correct amount of bran to add to food. This was the question of teaspoons and tablespoons. Even though thousands of cookbooks recommend a teaspoon of this or a tablespoon of that, there is surprisingly little information available as to what a teaspoon really is and what a tablespoon is. If you use water as a measuring medium and check your tablespoons against those of your neighbors, you will probably find that the amounts contained vary considerably.

The types of measuring teaspoon and tablespoon that are found in the housewares section of a department store should be more accurate, but I decided to check them. I was very surprised to find that they varied too. I purchased four different sets of measuring spoons, all of which differed in appearance. Two sets were plastic and two were metal. With an accurate chemical balance, using bran as the substance to be measured, I did a series of careful weighings to determine whether different brands of measuring spoons hold the same quantity of bran. I checked each of the four brands in both the teaspoon and tablespoon sizes against each other and carefully recorded the results.

A detailed analysis of this entire procedure is provided in Appendix C. After my research, I developed a standard to be used throughout this book:

Bran Flakes:
· 1 heaping teaspoon of bran weighs 2.3 grams and contains 0.3 grams of fiber.

· 1 heaping tablespoon of bran weighs 6.7 grams and contains 0.8 grams of fiber.

Fine Bran:
· 1 heaping teaspoon of fine bran weighs 4.6 grams, and contains 0.6 grams of fiber.
· 1 heaping tablespoon of fine bran weighs 9.0 grams and contains 1.1 grams of fiber.

Before you write to tell me that there are three teaspoons in a tablespoon and that my tablespoon figures are not exactly three times my teaspoon figures, let me assure you that I am aware of this. However, it does not hold true when you are dealing with *heaping* teaspoons and tablespoons, since the actual shape of the spoon determines the size and height of the mound of material that it will hold.

EAT FIBER WITH EACH MEAL

Now that I have recommended that you eat a minimum of 7 grams of fiber daily, preferably in the form of nine tablespoons of bran flakes or six tablespoons of finely ground bran, I must answer some inevitable questions. "Doctor, can I take in all nine tablespoons for breakfast and get it over with for the day?" Or, "Since I only have a cup of coffee for breakfast and lunch is a hamburger on the run, can I wait for dinner and take in all my fiber then?" Or, "I'm a busy executive. How am I going to have my three heaping tablespoons of bran flakes in bouillon at lunch? Even if I find a restaurant that will serve me a cup of broth, what do I do then? Do I take a small sack of bran out of my pocket and dump in three tablespoons?"

There are reasonably easy answers to these questions, but coming up with them was not easy. We live in a society that has evolved a lifestyle nutritionally detrimental to us. Our institutions, our supermarkets, our restaurants are not geared to the needs of the individual who is trying to improve his or her eating habits. While I will offer you a variety of ways to succeed, it is no secret that trying to eat properly is like swimming against the mainstream—you have to be persistent if you're going to succeed.

If many of this book's readers are persistent, this program should become part of a group effort. Then some of our institutions will adapt to the fiber needs of this new, enlightened group, and the task will become considerably easier for others. Once that happens, the enlightened group can grow more rapidly and become a sizable segment of the public, perhaps even a majority. The food suppliers will realize not only on what side their bread is buttered, but also that it should be buttered on whole wheat bread—and a proliferation of high-fiber foods will be assured.

In the meantime, it will take some effort to get your ration of fiber at lunch, though breakfast and dinner should be easy. When I'm confronted with a task that I expect to be difficult, I say to myself, "I often do things that are hard." Then I realize that I usually succeed at them. So, rather than agonizing over the hurdles of adding fiber to your diet, let's get right down to basics and see how to incorporate fiber into each meal.

Breakfast. Bran, being a cereal product, fits in very nicely with breakfast. The gung-ho health faddist probably will have no difficulty in swallowing three heaping tablespoons of bran, or even a full cup, and he or she won't care whether it's floating in water, or if he eats it dry. For most of us, however, eating straight bran or drinking it in a glass of water is not desirable. It is not that the flavor is bad, for indeed it has very little flavor, and what is there is quite pleasant. Rather, it has a feel, a texture that is unfamiliar to most of us.

A few people will report that they have tried it dry or in a glass of water, and that it tastes like straw, even though they have never tasted straw. The truth of the matter is that it tastes fibrous. It does not readily dissolve in the saliva and form a creamy goo like hollandaise sauce. It tastes like food, and it will remain in your mouth much longer than hollandaise sauce because it requires some chewing and further moistening before you feel like swallowing it.

Since most of you will not want to take it straight, you will mix it with another cereal in order to disguise it. With what? There are several choices. There is a new breed of breakfast cereal on the market, put out by several of the large manufacturers. These are not the flaky, highly processed, defibered breakfast cereals that have been popular for years. Rather, they are an attempt to give us a more natural product, and are certainly a step in the right direction. The basic ingredient of most of them is oats. To this is often added dried fruits such as figs or dates, coconut, raisins, and perhaps nuts. When mixed with milk they make a hardy, rather crunchy and filling breakfast. Some of the brand names are Country Morning, Quaker's 100% Natural, and Nature Valley Granola.

I am almost happy with these "natural cereals," but not quite. Because they were designed for a conditioned mass market of refined-food eaters, their product-design experts automatically decided to sweeten them. Some use sugar, some use brown sugar, and some use honey. This is their fatal flaw, but since they are easily available and are good in other ways, I will recommend their limited use.

Use them only to flavor the bran flakes. Therefore, use a minimum amount. One heaping tablespoon of any of them should be sufficient to flavor three heaping tablespoons of bran flakes. Add to this skim milk and you have a tasty breakfast.

If at first you find this cereal not sweet enough for your conditioned tastes, supplement the flavor with artificial sweetener. I recommend these sweeteners to my patients because I think they are very useful and I have seen no reasonable evidence of their being harmful. I particularly like the type that are mixtures, which have a few calories but are much more palatable. There is a list of many of these in Chapter 11.

(There are a number of "natural food" eaters in this country who will not eat either sugar or artificial sweeteners. I have formulated a special set of rules for these people, specifying the amount of honey or molasses they may use for a sweetener; these rules are listed on pp. 117–119.)

If you want to do something even better for yourself, go to a health-food store and look at the "granola" products. Granola is a generic term for a variety of mixed cereal products. Most health-food stores will have several of these, and they are usually refrigerated because they lack artificial preservatives.

It's important that you read the ingredients' label on each bag or box of health-food store granola. What you are searching for is one that has no sugar, whether it be white, natural, brown, or honey. Admittedly, these granolas are not as sweet as the very popular products mentioned above, but they are still tasty. They also have the advantage of avoiding the villainous sugar.

You may use more of this unsweetened granola—two or three heaping tablespoons—to mix with your bran flakes, and sweeten this with artificial sweetener, if you use it. To improve the granola's formula, you may add small amounts of raisins, nuts, or coconut shreds. The coconut should be the unsweetened variety, which I have only been able to find in health-food stores, rather than the kind you usually find in supermarkets.

Another cereal that contains no sugar—incidentally, one of the few unsweetened types that can be found in supermarkets—is Grape-Nuts (not flakes). It mixes well with bran.

An alternate breakfast is our all-around bran-buckwheat, one-to-three mixture mentioned in the previous chapter. This should probably be precooked in a larger batch and stored in your refrigerator. For breakfast heat up seven heaping tablespoons. When I eat this I add a little skim milk and sprinkle it with sugar substitute. I think it's a fantastic hot breakfast. If you want to beef it up you can drop a few raisins and nuts into it.

As for other conventional breakfast items, they are fine. You may have eggs, bacon, or ham. For toast, use whole wheat bread. You may have fruit, but if you're thinking of fruit juice, first study the C/F tables carefully. Rules presented later in this chapter will show that you can have orange juice if you add one heaping teaspoon of fine bran and stir it well.

In Chapter 11 you will find more suggestions for breakfast. These are concoctions of bran with other fibrous foods. Now that you know the principle, put your imagination to work. You can enjoy a variety of breakfasts that will each do their part to help you maintain your weight and keep you healthy.

Lunch. If you are one of the millions of people who work and have your lunch away from home, you've got a problem. How are you going to get the local hamburger-and-french-fries factory to supply you a high-fiber lunch? You can ask restaurants to include something satisfactory on the menu, but unless there are enough voices demanding better nutrition, you're not likely to have much success. Eventually, if enough people keep demanding, we will accomplish our goal, but your problem has to be solved right now.

You might object. You may say that lunch, five days a week, will be the exception. You may tell yourself that you will increase the amount of fiber at breakfast and dinner, thus still getting your 7 extra grams a day, and that will be just as good. But it is not as good. Without fiber for lunch you will be putting constipating, high-calorie meals into your digestive system.

You need fiber with every meal. There is no other way that is equally good. As we have each learned in our own life, if you want to do something badly enough, you find a way that works.

Here is the solution that works for me, personally. I take a small, one-pint thermos to work each day. It contains one cup of hot broth made from a bouillon cube and seven heaping tablespoons of the buckwheat-bran mixture, or three heaping tablespoons of bran alone. When lunchtime comes, I gobble it down (I also bring a plastic spoon with me) and then I go out for lunch. Sometimes after the soup I don't even want lunch, so I skip it. (You'll be amazed at how filling it is.) Is it good? I think it's great. I may be prejudiced because I know how good it is for me, but I think you'll agree that it's probably better than a soup you might get in a restaurant at lunch.

After you've had your fiber, all that is necessary is to use good judgment when ordering in the restaurant. You've already had your minimum lunchtime ration of fiber, but you don't have to stop with the minimum. But you may still run into trouble. You also know that white flour is forbidden, and therefore so is white bread and white buns. Since the sandwich is such a convenient lunch, I recommend that you attempt to find a place that serves sandwiches on whole wheat bread. The whole wheat bread they serve may not be the most desirable, but it will be better than white bread.

Or you and a few friends could request that a favorite restaurant stock whole wheat bread. If it agrees, you can have virtually any kind of sandwich for lunch. If all this seems like too much of a bother to you, then I will reply that sometimes living is a bother. Here we are talking about procedures that may preserve your life. Is that too much of a bother?

Later I am going to talk about a concerted effort to make restauranteurs change their ways. A group effort could accomplish this, particularly since I am not asking them to make many changes. Ninety-five percent of their menu can stay the same. Isn't it amazing that a few high-fiber dishes, soups, and vegetables can make such a big difference?

I feel a great victory will be won when the large hamburger chains offer an optional whole wheat bun on their menu.

There is a second alternative for lunch that I have used many times, on days when I did not bring soup to the office. It is possible to go to a restaurant and get a cup of soup or broth, but it is unlikely there will be bran for you to put in it. I have gone into restaurants many times carrying a little vial or small plastic bag containing two heaping tablespoons of fine bran or three heaping tablespoons of bran flakes, dumped it in the soup, and then proceeded to enjoy my lunch. Admittedly, at times I have had to face inquisitive glances when I have been observed clandestinely dropping this beige powder into my food, but I have as yet never been arrested, and until I am I shall continue to do this.

So that I am never without my bran, I keep a number of vials of it in my desk at the office. Two tablespoons of fine bran are in each vial, and when I have to go out for lunch, I take one with me.

If you are one of those people who eat your lunch at home, in your own kitchen, there is no problem. You can either have your bran in broth, as a prelude to the meal, or you can incorporate it into the lunch. However, whether you are a dieter or not, I prefer that you have it before the meal in broth, because it serves an extra purpose. If you have your broth fifteen minutes before eating the rest of the meal, and in that interval drink one glass of water (8 ounces), it will serve as an appetite depressant that will definitely limit your intake of the rest of the meal. It may even substitute for the meal.

I think once you have formed the broth habit it will become as routine as brushing your teeth. Having broth before the meal is the easiest way to keep your proper weight, once you have reached it. But if soup before lunch becomes monotonous, then sometimes have your quota of bran mixed in your food.

What lunchtime foods can you mix bran into? How about in mashed potatoes? What kind of a book on weight control tells you to eat mashed potatoes? "Why, I haven't eaten mashed potatoes in years," you might say. "Yum!" It's permitted as long as it fulfills the requirement of being less than 100 on the carbohydrate-fiber ratio chart. It's how you prepare the potatoes that counts. Here's the hard way. Boil up the bran in a small amount of water for about ten minutes, while your potatoes are cooking in another pot. Then mash or whip the bran into your potatoes. This is the biggest improvement in mashed potatoes in two thousand years.

Now, here's the easy way to make mashed potatoes. Use one of the powdered or flaky mashed potato mixes. These are essentially dehydrated potatoes, and are not refined to the extent that we process wheat. They are simple to use and not at all bad to taste. You'll have to modify the recipe a bit. You'll need about 50 percent more water than is called for on the box, and you'll have to boil the bran in the water for about ten minutes first. But the result is great.

Here are some super-duper variations. Mix some chopped, boiled onions in with your brown mashed potatoes. Wow! Or, when boiling the potatoes, leave the skins on and leave lots of small pieces of cooked potato skin in the mashed potatoes. Do they add flavor and vitamins!

Where else can you add bran? Mix the ground beef with moistened bran flakes in almost any proportion. The more bran the better. But remember, the bran absorbs fluid and the mixture can become dry. Don't hesitate to add water to the hamburger-bran mix. It will improve it greatly. Season your hamburgers and fry or broil them as usual. Or you can also mix the buckwheat-bran combo in your hamburger. Try them both, experiment, see which you like best. When mixed with meat, you won't even notice any difference in texture. You're probably already accustomed to hamburger mixed with vegetable protein extenders. When you add fiber to this dish you're really doing yourself a favor, because you're not only getting the benefits of the fiber, but you're cutting way down on the animal fats, which are quite high in calories.

How about meat loaf? Great! Experiment, invent, but no more bread crumbs in it, no more soaked bread. From the standpoint of taste alone, you're going to like the bran better.

Tuna fish salad, chicken salad, turkey salad, and egg salad? Yup. Remember, you are only restricting your intake of refined sugar and flour. You may have everything else.

Of course, a sandwich at home is great for lunch—as long as it is on whole wheat bread. The commercially available, packaged whole wheat breads can be used, but they're not nearly as good as some of those made by small bakeries or those found in health-food stores. Preferable to any of them is my Perfectly Healthy Bread, found in Chapter 11. True, making bread is a lot of work, but what a reward. If you make several extra loaves you can freeze them for later use.

Once you get into the swing of things and develop a routine for including fiber with your lunch, you will find it is a very easy part of preparing your meal. You will quickly get used to the small number of simple changes I am asking you to make. Whether you eat out or at home, your new diet will run smoothly.

Dinner. Now we come to dinner. For most of us, this is the high point of the eating experience. All that I have said about breakfast and lunch applies doubly to dinner. Have your three heaping tablespoons of bran either as a prelude or with dinner. Because we generally eat more at dinner than any other meal, try to exceed the basic three tablespoon requirement by incorporating fiber into the various foods you eat. It will accrue to your benefit.

Take the time to study the carbohydrate-fiber ratio tables in Chapter 12. Have a pad of paper and pencil at hand. You will get some good ideas and you will probably include some delicious foods in your dinners that heretofore you have ignored.

One good example is spaghetti. "Spaghetti! I don't believe it, he's going to let me eat spaghetti!" Wait until you taste my spaghetti sauce (Chapter 11). It's delicious! I'm not going to have any trouble convincing Italian families to make this one when they see how it will cut their meat costs. Of course, the spaghetti itself, the pasta, is still a problem, but would you believe that I have found spaghetti and lasagna noodles made with whole wheat flour in the health-food stores, and they're great! They are more chewy, the way I like them. True "al dente."

Fried chicken or fried fish? Absolutely. Guess what you're going to "bread" them with? You guessed right. You'll find out how in the recipe section.

I also have a recipe for natural gravy. You'll learn how to turn natural gravy into one unusually delicious and high in fiber.

The nicest part of a high-fiber diet is that you can see you are taking very positive steps toward maintaining your weight and enjoying good health without having to endure some odd-ball diet. In fact, as you will see for yourself, meals fortified with fiber do not appear appreciably different from your present diet so rich in naked calories. Even from the start you will probably not have any feeling of being on a diet.

For dinner you can have the usual multi-course meal. If you choose soup as a first course, you can use the bouillon or broth already discussed, or you can incorporate bran into any other soup that meets my specifications.

If your main course is one of the animal protein foods—meat, fowl or fish—there are a number of ways to combine them with bran or other fiber foods. Bran mixes well with dishes in which the animal protein food is chopped, ground, or diced. It fits in very well with beef stew, tuna fish salad, or chicken croquettes. Check Chapter 11 for some great sauces, gravies, and dressings that are quite high in fiber.

After telling you that you can incorporate fiber into virtually anything you eat, I must remind you not to get carried away. It is true that you should eat as much fiber as possible, but it isn't necessary for each mouthful to contain fiber. It is only necessary that each mouthful of carbohydrate-containing food contains fiber, and that each meal has its quota of fiber. There is a very simple rule you can follow to make your calculations easier: if all the carbohydrate-containing foods you eat have a C/F of less than 100, then every mouthful of *carbohydrate* you eat will automatically contain some fiber. If you want to eat a plant food that has a C/F of more than 100, add fiber in the form of bran to it so that its C/F is lowered to below 100. Generally this will mean adding one heaping teaspoon of bran per serving to this food. By following this rule, every mouthful of carbohydrate-containing food will contain fiber, and you will not be eating any naked calories.

If you prefer to eat a steak "right off the hoof" instead of ground beef mixed with fiber, don't feel guilty about it. As long as the rest of the meal provides the fiber, and as long as every mouthful of plant food has its fiber, you are doing the right thing.

Vegetables adapt very well to bran or other fibrous materials such as sesame seeds or coconut. I have already spoken of potatoes, but green, yellow, and white vegetables are discussed in the recipe section. You may have bread with your dinner as long as it satisfies the requirements of the carbohydrate-fiber ratio, which means that it is whole wheat. Dessert? Well, concentrate on fruits, although there are other suggestions in Chapter 11.

To sum up, you should have fiber with every meal. You cannot correct an omission by doubling up at the next meal. By then, the naked calories are already deep inside your digestive system, slowing your digestive process, constipating your system, and feeding your body excess calories.

The best solution for most of you is to maintain your present diet, eliminate only refined carbohydrates, and find easy ways to add the fiber you need to every meal. This is a reasonable and simple change, yet it will make a world of difference to your health and weight.

Don't forget to introduce fiber to your diet over a two-week period, as spelled out in Chapter 6.

As you learn how to include bran in your cooking, you will probably experiment and try new recipes, not only those provided in the recipe section. Most of your favorite recipes and "family specials" can be easily adapted to this diet simply by adding fiber to their ingredients. In almost every case, added fiber won't make any difference in your enjoyment of a food.

If you come up with anything spectacular, please write me and tell me about it. My address is given in Chapter 9. It's important to share your recipes with others, as I'm sharing mine with you, because the benefits of this diet are so dramatic.

PUBLIC ENEMIES #1 AND #2: REFINED SUGAR AND WHITE FLOUR

I demand that you do your best to avoid Public Enemy #1, refined sugar, and Public Enemy #2, white flour.

Public Enemy #1 comes in many disguises. It may appear in any shade, from dark brown to lily white. Sugar may pose as a seductive woman in the form of a smooth liquid honey just to confuse you, or it may hide by trying to get lost in the midst of a crowd of otherwise respectable foods. But don't be fooled. Sugar is your enemy and you are making war on it.

Although I believe sugar is addictive, I have no scientific data to substantiate my beliefs. But seventeen years in practice observing sugar-eating patients must be worth something. The overindulgence in sugar consumption is unbelievable. There are patients who tell me that they don't stop eating until they vomit. In my own case I've noted that it's the first piece of candy that's fatal. I can do without sweets, but once I have the first piece, it's almost impossible to stop. How many patients have told me that they intended to have only one thin sliver of cake and ended up eating the entire thing!

How many office workers literally live for that mid-morning doughnut and coffee break? How many people can't watch a movie without a bag of candy in the lap?

However, after speaking to thousands of patients, I have not found this to be true with honey and molasses. I am still opposed to their use in any significant quantity, but I recognize that they are a shade better than white and brown sugar on the scale of evil. I have never had a patient report to me that he or she was a honey addict. There is apparently something self-limiting in honey and molasses. After eating a small amount there does not seem to be that strong a desire for more. As a result, I will permit the minimal use of honey and molasses by those people who are prejudiced against artificial sweeteners.

Public Enemy #2, white flour, is also good at disguises, but its most fearsome threats are in white bread and the seductive clothes it wears in pastries, cakes, pies, Danish, and other sweets. Some of these can be made with whole wheat flour, and we heartily approve. But that slice of devil's food cake with thick chocolate frosting is taboo!

You will frequently find sugar and flour on the list of ingredients of prepared packaged foods such as canned soups. It's unfortunate that many canned and packaged foods do contain small amounts of sugar, flour, dextrose, sucrose, cornstarch, etc. These prepared products would often be perfectly acceptable if they did not include these refined carbohydrates.

After stating so emphatically that sugar and white flour are dangerous substances and should not be part of the human diet, it might seem inconsistent to now tell you that you may eat a small amount of them in a few canned and packaged foods.

Many people are not aware that the federal government requires food manufacturers to list the ingredients contained within their product in the decreasing order of the amount present. These lists are usually in very tiny print on the bottom of the back or side labels of most products. In these lists, the item listed first is present in the greatest quantity, and the item listed last is present in the smallest quantity. Even though the label does not tell you the exact amount of any ingredient, the order of the ingredients lets you make a reasonable guess of the approximate amount.

For example, a popular bean with bacon soup has a list of ingredients something like this: cooked pea beans, water, tomatoes, bacon, carrots, salt, celery, beef fat, sugar, corn starch, monosodium glutamate, and flavorings. The objectionable items are sugar and corn starch, but notice where they are placed on the list. Except for the seasonings they fall last. There is less of each of them than there is of beef fat. Once you prepare the soup the amount of fat is generally visible floating on the top. This gives you an idea that there is a very small amount of fat and that therefore the sugar and corn starch are present in even smaller quantities. This soup would be acceptable on The Weight-Maintenance Diet only because its refined carbohydrates are present in such small amounts. One can of soup will usually serve two people. As specified in my rules, you should add two teaspoons of finely ground bran or one tablespoon of bran flakes to alter the soup's carbohydrate-fiber ratio.

Another exception to my "no refined sugar or flour" rule might be the case where you are using a packaged product that is so small to begin with that regardless of the order of ingredients, it cannot have much effect on you. A dry powdered gravy mix that I often use contains only 21 grams of powder. Here the ingredients are relatively unimportant, since when I prepare it I combine this powder with much greater quantities of other foods, including at least one heaping tablespoon of bran, and thus the final gravy contains very little refined carbohydrates.

Your naked calorie war, just like any war, will rely on your intelligence department to give you the information you need to win. Let your intelligence ferret out the enemy on the ingredients' labels of food, so that you avoid excessive consumption of refined carbohydrates.

Always read the labels! They tell you what is in the food you eat. They tell you whether you are being nourished or poisoned. If you eat something you are not supposed to, it's your fault too, not just the manufacturers'.

Exactly how cautious should you be? The complete omission of sugar and white flour from your diet should be your goal, but this is obviously an ideal. Try to unmask and eliminate the naked calorie to whatever extent you can. If you do not reach 100 percent compliance, whatever naked calories you have eliminated will work to your benefit.

So that you know when to stop, I have formulated the following rules. If you can go "all the way" and kick those naked calories out the door forever, you are doing yourself a big favor. But if you can't accomplish this and must have some sweets in your life, the following rules will show you how to include these sweets with minimal impact on your health.

By observing these rules, your food may contain a small number of naked calories, which you will cover with bran—and this opens up to you many more foods in the supermarket. But remember, you have been given a *limited* license to eat a wider variety of foods. Make sure that the sugar in them is a *minor* ingredient. Use your judgment, and be careful!

Rules for Using Refined Carbohydrates on The Weight-Maintenance Diet *

1. Sugar (both white and brown sugar) should not be used in any of the foods you prepare at home.
2. You can use a small amount of honey or molasses as a sweetener in your home cooking, but these must not provide more than 5 percent of the calories present in the final food.

For example, if you bake oatmeal cookies and choose to use honey instead of artificial sweetener, the amount of calories the honey provides must be less than 5 percent of the total number of calories in each cookie.

For those who will use some artificial sweetener, Chapter 11 explains how to make a mixture of honey and artificial sweetener. This lets you use a minimum amount of artificial sweetener and a minimum amount of honey at the same time. You will be able to use this sweetening mixture in a wide variety of home-cooked foods.

3. As I mentioned before, your biggest problem will not be in baking, but in buying prepared products in the super-market. Food manufacturers do not state the exact quantity

---

* Shortly I will discuss the use of artificial sweeteners. For many people they are the answer to the need for sweetening. Those who object to the use of artificial sweeteners are in a serious dilemma. It is for them that these rules have been provided.

of their ingredients. In most cases you will have to read the label and make an intelligent guess.

If the sugar listed on the label is a minor ingredient, add one teaspoon of bran to make the food permissible to eat. However, if sugar is a major ingredient, don't buy the product.

At the present time I am planning a concerted effort to collect data on the sugar and refined carbohydrate content of popular mass-market foods. I intend to secure this data by the voluntary compliance of manufacturers. I will be shocked if I find that manufacturers are not willing to divulge this information, which would be in the public's interest. The public has an obvious right to know what it is eating. This data will be the subject of a future book. Until this research is done and the book is written, you will have to read the labels and guess.

4. When you add honey to home-cooked foods or consume sugar in a packaged food, you must lower the carbohydrate-fiber ratio by adding bran. In most cases one or two extra heaping teaspoons per serving (depending on how much sugar or honey is present) will be sufficient.

5. You do not have to judge the inclusion of refined flour as critically as that of sugar. If the amount is rather small or if the flour is used, for example, to thicken the product, it is allowed, providing you add extra bran.

When, however, the product is predominantly white flour, such as in baked goods, breads, etc., it is never permitted.

6. For those people who do not object, artificial sweeteners can be substituted for even the small amount of honey permitted. A number of artificial sweeteners available at your supermarket are suitable for baking. Both Sweet 'n Low and the new, granulated Sucaryl will not denature during cooking. In fact, they withstand approximately the same range of cooking temperatures as sugar. I have tested this myself, and everything I have baked with these artificial sweeteners has

tasted delicious. There probably are other products that will work just as well. There is no taste excuse for using sugar or honey in baking. If you find artificial sweeteners acceptable, they are all you need to use.

7. Perhaps the most important deviation I will permit is in whole wheat bread, since I consider bread to be a very important part of the diet. Most breads are not particularly palatable unless they contain a small amount of sweetening, even though it is not apparent that they are sweet. Almost all commercial breads, including whole wheat bread, contain sugar.

You will note in the recipe section that my Perfectly Healthy Bread is an example of the use of artificial sweetener to produce a wonderful result. I developed this recipe and it is the only one I have ever seen for bread with artificial sweetener. I can immodestly say that it is the best bread I have ever eaten. Its good taste, combined with its C/F of 20, makes Perfectly Healthy Bread not only acceptable but extremely desirable.

Remember, no packaged white bread meets my specifications when it comes to the C/F. The better whole wheat breads, in spite of their containing a small amount of sugar, are acceptable.

One last warning. Despite its use in the title of this book, don't be fooled by the word natural, especially when it is applied to honey or molasses. The world is full of natural poisons. The hemlock that dispatched Socrates from the earth was natural, and the venom in a rattlesnake bite is natural also. Your shampoo and your soap might be made of natural ingredients, but you're not having them for dinner tonight. The word natural can easily be used to fool you. Look at honey. Did you ever wonder why busy bees are so busy? Well, I'll tell you. They are busy refining sugar.

ARTIFICIAL SWEETENERS

Admittedly, a lifetime addiction to sugar is not easily shaken. You "sugar junkies" can try beating it "cold turkey," if I may use these phrases, but I have no medical objection to substituting reasonable amounts of artificial sweeteners. I have looked carefully at the evidence on artificial sweeteners, and I have seen no concrete evidence that they are harmful.

At present, the majority of artificial sweeteners rely on saccharin for their sweetening power. The major objection seems to be the "bitter after-taste" that a few people report. Many people report, however, and almost all my patients who try artificial sweeteners are included, that a taste for artificial sweeteners is quickly acquired. After using them for a short while they become fully acceptable.

There is a relatively new breed of artificial sweetener on the market that is usually saccharin in conjunction with a very small amount of calories containing sugar. The naked calories in these are minimal, and these products are acceptable. By our taste comparisons, they take the blue ribbon. Some of them are Sweet 'n Low, Sugar Twin, and granulated Sucaryl, but there are many others.

By the time this book reaches the bookstore, it is possible that a new kind of sweetener, now being tested, will have been introduced to the market. Advance information on this product is very encouraging. It looks, pours, and measures just like sugar, and I hope that since it is made of amino acids, which are completely natural substances, it will prove to be the perfect substitute for sugar. This may be the product the people who object to artificial sweeteners have been waiting for.

VITAMINS

If you follow my advice, you will eat a well-balanced diet fortified with fiber, omitting only sugar and white flour. Chances are that vitamin deficiencies will not be a problem. If, however, you don't make a detailed analysis of your total intake of food, you can't be 100 percent certain.

My inclination is to play safe. If you take a single multiple-vitamin tablet every day, odds are that you won't have problems with vitamin deficiencies. What kind should you take? It should contain the recommended daily allowances (RDA) recognized by the United States government. You don't need the high-potency "therapeutic" powerhouse that sells for the top price.

What about the vitamins you are going to miss by not eating "enriched" white bread or by omitting honey from cooking? It should give you little solace to know that the poison you've just taken also contains small amounts of things that are actually good for you. When these foods are weighed on the scale of health, they are not only lightweights, but the evidence says that they are downright destructive.

FLUIDS

For good health, fluids are desirable. Perhaps the most desirable, indeed, the most necessary, is water. Water in itself is not harmful and it is unlikely that anyone could drink a quantity that would be considered harmful. Water does not cause you to gain weight or keep you from losing it.

Most of the fluids you drink consist of water flavored with relatively small amounts of other substances. This is true for both hot drinks such as coffee, tea, and cocoa, and for cold drinks such as soda, iced tea, and fruit juices.

In general, the fibrous foods you eat swell by absorbing amounts of water much greater than their own weight. These water-swollen fibers contribute a great deal to the weight-maintenance and weight-loss phenomena reported in this book. I would like to see you drink a minimum of four full eight-ounce glasses of water a day. One of these should be taken approximately fifteen minutes after each meal. (Other beverages besides water are acceptable.) You should reserve the fourth glass for bedtime. These four glasses of water, or other beverages, should be in addition to all the other fluids you consume during the day.

If you seem to retain water—that is, if you have edema (swelling)—you should consult your physician because you have other problems, perhaps serious ones. The water itself is not the cause of the problem.

While I'm on the subject of physicians, remember that I insist you consult your physician first, before you embark on a lifetime dietary program. I have several reasons for this. For one thing, he or she may know something special about you that I couldn't possibly guess. Secondly, it's a great excuse for getting you to have a physical examination, for which you are probably overdue anyway. Third and most important, it will call your physician's attention to the subject of the naked calorie. From my own experience I have found that most family physicians are still relatively unaware of "the fiber story," although more and more articles on this subject are appearing in the medical literature your family doctor reads. I would genuinely welcome inquiries from him or her. My address for correspondence is given in Chapter 9.

EXERCISE

The importance of exercise for weight maintenance is significant enough to fill a book. As a matter of fact, it has already filled many books. I am very much in favor of exercise as part of this diet.

The vast majority of persons who read this book will not be adversely affected by exercise, no matter how strenuous, if they approach it gradually and sensibly. There may be some people, however, with severe medical problems who truly should not exercise. There is no way I can tell you in which category you belong. If there is any question, consult your family doctor and heed his or her advice.

What system of exercise should you follow? I believe that the more you exercise, the better it is for you. In my medical practice I have tried to encourage my patients to burn calories. The number of calories that are burned is proportional to the effort expended. The exercise that leaves you thoroughly tired and momentarily winded is the one that does you the most good. Don't be afraid of becoming winded. Indeed, that should be your goal.

An excellent program that deals with this subject is available in the books written by Dr. Kenneth H. Cooper on the subject of aerobics. I have long advocated their use. Dr. Cooper has tried to utilize scientific parameters to answer the question of how much exercise you need, and he endeavors to answer that question in specific terms.

There are other excellent books on this subject, but it is not necessary to follow an exercise system. One of the best ways to exercise is by doing something that is fun. Sports are perfect. I try to play some tennis every day. Even though I don't rate myself as being particularly skillful, it's nice to know that something that is so much fun is also good for me.

Another book well worth reading on this subject is *Energetics* by Grant Gwinup. Here the author attempts to define the number of calories burned up by various forms of physical activity. This could prove very useful to you in estimating how many calories you use up per day. Bear in mind that every calorie you burn through exercise counterbalances that many calories you have eaten.

I hope you do not have the impression that because I have given so little space to exercise I do not consider it vitally important. I have not discussed this to the extent that it deserves because I am anxious to get across the new ideas contained in this book. Therefore, don't minimize the importance of exercise. Get out there and sweat a little! It will do you good!

CHAPTER 8

THE EAT-ENOUGH, HIGH-FIBER REDUCING DIET

The High-Fiber Reducing Diet incorporates the same basic principles as The Weight-Maintenance Diet. Eat a minimum of 10 to 12 grams of fiber daily and eliminate all refined carbohydrates. While this sounds like a simple change, it is a major step forward in the quality of the food you eat. With only a small variation from your usual habits, you have returned to nutritional normalcy.

Unfortunately, these two nutritional basics are abnormal in our present society, because you are not provided automatic access to fibrous foods. In the reducing diet, as in the maintenance diet, you must make an extra effort to purchase additional dietary fiber and include it in your meals.

Now that you have followed the medical evidence and learned what a normal diet really should be, you can see why I believe that the cause of the major problem of obesity faced by all industrialized countries is that you are eating naked calories and fiber-free diets. This forces too many digestible calories into your body, where they crawl through you at constipation speed. These refined diets put pounds on you and make you forfeit the good health and easy weight control that would be yours if you were eating adequate amounts of fiber.

Since The Weight-Maintenance Diet automatically regulates the amount of calories your body receives, it alone can produce a gradual loss of weight in overweight people. If it were adopted and employed religiously by those who are obese, it would eventually return them to a sensible weight. But this would be a very slow process and it would take a long time.

In my medical practice I see the damage obesity causes every day. To put it bluntly, if you are overweight you are in a critical situation, and you cannot afford to wait while The Weight-Maintenance Diet slowly brings your weight under control. Strong, indeed lifesaving measures are needed. I pray that you heed this warning and follow the recommendations of this chapter if you are overweight.

The cornerstone of The High-Fiber Reducing Diet is the daily minimum intake of fiber. This added fiber will have these three goals:

1. Because of its bulk and its ability to absorb fluid, it will satisfy your hunger and depress your appetite for higher calorie foods.

2. The fiber will decrease the transit time of food through the intestinal tract, thus lowering the number of calories your body receives from the food you eat.

3. By restoring the balance of your food to the part-fiber, part-nutrient composition it should be, your digestive system will begin to return to its normal working order, and you will reduce your chances of contracting a wide variety of diseases.

In the reducing diet I will make the same recommendation for the minimum daily intake of fiber as in The Weight-Maintenance Diet. There are two additions: first, underline the word *minimum,* and second, do not ever miss this added fiber in any meal. This means that faithfully, three times a day, you must have at least three heaping tablespoons of fiber added to your meals.

You may think it unusual to use a diet that tells you not to miss a single meal. With most diets, if you skip a meal and get fewer calories as a result, that's great! With this diet, I am making sure you eat properly. Believe me, it will make your whole weight-loss program much more successful if you eat every meal.

Some fiber should be taken before dinner in a broth, to serve as an appetite depressant. However, this applies only at dinner. In the case of breakfast and lunch, the fiber portion will be the entire meal; you may eat more than my recommended minimum.

Your extra fiber from bran should be distributed fairly equally at all three meals. This is easily done by taking three heaping tablespoons of bran flakes and adding it to some other substance. Usually, you will add it to a liquid such as milk with cereal, in broth, or in gravies, casseroles, or mixed in other dishes.

On this High-Fiber Reducing Diet, your breakfast will usually consist of a very high-fiber cereal only, or occasionally a low-calorie egg substitute, and you must not skip it. Lunch will be rather simple and quite low calorie. Dinner will be liberal and will prove quite adequate. Your "real" meal will be dinner, although, depending on your schedule and lifestyle, you may interchange lunch and dinner. Of course, no refined carbohydrates will be allowed at any time.

You can eat an almost unlimited quantity of the type of dinner I suggest. One problem you will not have on this diet that you have on almost every other diet is the problem of getting up from the dinner table hungry. You will not be hungry here because you will be eating a rather large amount of food.

Any intake between meals should be of a very minimal nature, and an intake of fluid at meals and just after them will be required. I will set minimum requirements for fluids, but you should exceed them. It is desirable for you to have as much fluid as possible.

You will take advantage of every trick, gimmick, or scheme that can help you reach your proper weight. For instance, you will be encouraged to make full use of spices and other seasonings to make the diet more acceptable. You should also use abnormally large amounts of very low-calorie foods to fill yourself up, such as mushrooms in cooked dishes, or a snack of celery or cucumbers.

I will make specific recommendations as to how much meat, fish, eggs, etc., you may or must have during each week. If you follow my instructions to the letter, you will not be hungry, and therefore you will have no trouble sticking to the regime. If you do not stick to this reducing diet, it will not be the result of hunger.

You will have to use more individual judgment on The High-Fiber Reducing Diet than on The Weight-Maintenance Diet. On the reducing diet your breakfast and lunch are composed mostly of bran. Therefore, I cannot say that you already eat 3 to 5 grams of fiber a day, because the composition of both breakfast and lunch have been changed. Yet you still need 10 to 12 (preferably 12) grams of fiber a day.

This is where your judgment comes in. You will be using a bit of granola or another cereal to flavor your bran for breakfast, and this will provide some fiber. At lunch you will be permitted an open-faced sandwich on whole wheat bread, and this bread will provide some more fiber. Then, your dinner will contain some fiber.

Use the charts in Chapter 12 and estimate how much fiber you are getting. If you have not reached 10 to 12 grams of fiber for the day, add an extra heaping tablespoon of bran to both breakfast and lunch. You can estimate the additional amount of bran you need by using the tables in Appendix C, Amount of Fiber in Bran.

In other words, to reach your total minimum intake of 12 grams you may have to use as much as four heaping tablespoons of bran for breakfast and lunch, and three heaping tablespoons at dinner. If you are still short of 12 grams after this, add another heaping tablespoon, this time at dinner, to make the three meals equal.

When you add extra bran to my recommended three heaping tablespoons at each meal, spread it evenly among the three meals. I have recommended that you distribute it between breakfast and lunch first because your vegetables and salad at dinner will probably contain some fiber. But remember, your total amount of fiber should be taken fairly equally at your three meals.

If you do not remain with this diet and do not achieve your proper weight, I can only conclude that it is because you truly don't want to be thin. If you don't want to lose weight you should read no further. Everything in this chapter is intended for those who would like to become thin and stay thin. As I said before, you have freedom of choice, and you are the only one who can make this decision.

After seventeen years of watching a needless and depressing loss of human life because of obesity, I can only accept one excuse as valid, and that is hunger. If you follow my system you will not be hungry. If you choose to follow my system, and despite the lack of hunger still overeat and remain fat, it is your decision and you must live—and die—with it. Your choice, to be completely honest, is a life or death decision.

EAT THREE MEALS A DAY

You are to eat three meals a day and only three meals a day. You may not skip any of these meals, since each provides the vital fiber that you need.

Although I prefer that you do without it, I will permit a midmorning, a midafternoon, and a late-evening snack. If you can skip any of them, please do. Your midmorning and midafternoon snacks may only consist of something in the cucumber, pickle, or celery stalk category. Your late-night snack may consist of an apple or a pear. For those who have a serious late-night eating problem—if you are truly hungry—I recommend another cup of bouillon, but this time with somewhat less bran, two heaping tablespoons.

No naked calories or refined calories *at all* while you are reducing! You cannot afford a slip-up of any kind during the several weeks to several months you are dieting. You must regard a single slip as a crack in the dike. If it should occur, the crack must be sealed immediately, and you must see that no further slips occur.

Breakfast. The breakfasts given in The Weight-Maintenance Diet are quite satisfactory for this weight-reduction program. Three heaping tablespoons of bran flakes or two heaping table-spoons of fine bran are the minimum amount required. This is to be added to no more than one heaping tablespoon of an unrefined breakfast cereal. The cereal you use *must not contain any* sugar, molasses, or honey.

Where do you find it? In the supermarket you can buy Grape-Nuts or shredded wheat, both of which have no sugar, or you can find an acceptable granola in a health-food store. I usually eat health-food granolas. They meet my specifications if they are unsweetened. Be sure to check the ingredients label.

When you eat it, the cereal-bran mixture can be sweetened with a granular, artificial sweetener. (Honey is not permitted at all on the reducing diet.) Add just enough skim milk to make it edible, and that is your breakfast.

If you wish a hot breakfast, then the bran-buckwheat mixture described in Chapter 6 is absolutely delicious. It can be sweet-ened with artificial sweetener and a little skim milk can be added. You may also add the bran to hot cereal such as Whea-tena or Ralston.

One or two mornings a week you may have a low-calorie egg product that has recently been introduced to the market. It is called Second Nature. It is a liquid that comes in a small, milk-type carton. You will find it in the refrigerated section of the supermarket. When heated in a skillet, it simulates scrambled eggs or omelets. It has about half the calories of eggs with vir-tually no fat. This liquid can be mixed with fine bran and a little water before it is heated. But remember, no more often than twice a week.

Be careful of other egg replacements or substitutes that are not low calorie at all, but which have as their selling point the absence of cholesterol. Only *low-calorie* egg products are acceptable for your breakfast, and the only one I have found is Second Nature. There may be other types in other areas of the country.

If you wish to have a cup of coffee with artificial sweetener, it is all right. You may use no more than one ounce—two tablespoons—of skim milk in your coffee to lighten it. No cream, artificial cream, or dry powder cream substitute is permitted on the weight-reduction diet.

These breakfasts are quite filling and should easily satisfy your hunger until lunch. They are tasty and fulfill all the requirements of a good breakfast.

If you prefer a quicker breakfast, you may have juice instead of cereal. It must be tomato juice, with the bran mixed in. Six ounces of tomato juice containing three heaping tablespoons of bran flakes will be your breakfast. Actually, two heaping tablespoons of fine bran mixes better with juice. To beef it up, a dash of some spice, such as of Worcestershire, is permissible.

If you tell yourself that these breakfasts are dull and uninteresting, that you prefer waffles topped with syrup and bacon on the side, then you should also tell yourself—out loud for emphasis—"I prefer being fat, uncomfortable, unsightly, unhealthy, and dead."

Midmorning snack. I prefer that you don't have it, but if you insist, you may have a cucumber, a sour pickle, two stalks of celery, or as much as a dozen plump raw mushrooms. Yes, I did say raw mushrooms. They are an excellent diet food.

I was first introduced to raw mushrooms at cocktail parties, where they were used along with other raw vegetables as a vehicle to pick up high-calorie dips. The incongruity stuck in my mind. I was using this wonderful, low-calorie food as a utensil to shove high-calorie goo into my gullet. I was more impressed with the good flavor, chewability, and filling nature of the mushroom.

If anything comes closer than bran to being an ideal diet

food, it is the mushroom. Its only flaw is that it doesn't have the fiber, but do you know what else it doesn't have? It doesn't have carbohydrates, protein, or fat. In short, it is the closest thing to an edible nonfood that exists. If it weren't for the fact that you would develop severe malnutrition or other medical problems, you could stuff yourself with mushrooms all day long and still starve yourself.

I personally eat a considerable number of mushrooms. It's a shame they're so expensive. I buy mine wholesale in three-pound baskets, just like the supermarkets do. You might investigate this possibility where you live.

What do you do with raw mushrooms? You put salt and pepper on them. You put a little Worcestershire sauce on them. You dip them in mustard or ketchup. Lightly touch them to a little Marmite or Vegex which are flavorings explained more fully in Chapter 13.

In addition to mushrooms, celery, sour pickles or cucumbers, Chapter 11 lists other possible snack foods.

Lunch. The millions of overweight people who are forced to eat their lunches out have a problem. You cannot expect to convince restaurants overnight to include high-fiber soups and dishes on their menus. The most you can hope is that within a short time a few restaurants in each city will offer a few high-fiber dishes. Until this happens, it is up to you. Although the problem is difficult, it is not impossible.

There are two reasonably easy alternatives from which you can choose. First, you can brown bag it, that is, bring your lunch with you. Before you reject this possibility, consider whether it is really impossible, and weigh the inconvenience against the benefits. Does your boss always forbid eating lunch in the office, or would he or she listen if you made a special appeal? Would it really jeopardize your social position in the organization to bring your own lunch? How much money, per week, would you save? Would the loss of an hour's camaraderie with your buddies be more than you could bear? If so, I suggest you enlist them in this project. You could all enjoy your high-fiber lunch together.

Assuming that you can bring your lunch with you, I strongly recommend that you bring soup in a thermos jug. Soup is very easy to make. You can simply open a can or drop a bouillon cube in boiling water. Some of the bouillon products are very tasty, but different brands vary in quality, so do some testing.

To this soup add three or four heaping tablespoons of bran. The bran can be boiled in the soup for a few minutes to make it a bit softer, but this is not necessary. It is quite possible you won't be able to tell the difference. The bran gives the soup body. If you desire a lighter texture, you can use the finely ground bran, in which case only two heaping tablespoons will be necessary.

Lunch should only be one cup of soup. Since bran is surprisingly filling, you should be able to make this your entire lunch. If you choose other than a clear broth, I must insist that it be your entire lunch. Also, it should be obvious that on a reducing diet, you must not choose cream soups, potato soup, noodle, or rice soups.

If you feel you cannot get by on this (again, please don't make a prejudgment since bran makes the soup much more filling than you think), then I will permit some additional food. Since you are bringing lunch from home, one open-faced sandwich is permitted. The bread must be whole wheat and only one slice. You could use this one slice of bread to make a closed, half-sandwich. One brand of packaged whole wheat bread is very thinly sliced, so two slices are approximately the same as one regular slice. You may have lean roast beef, turkey, or chicken, but, without counting calories, be reasonable as to the quantity. You may not have *any* processed luncheon meats.

You may drink tea or coffee with artificial sweetener, diet sodas, or plain water with your lunch.

Regardless of how much food you have for lunch, ten to fifteen minutes later drink an eight-ounce glass of water or one of the other beverages.

The second alternative for lunch is the one I suggested in The Weight-Maintenance Diet for the days when you do not bring soup to work. You can go to a restaurant and get a cup of clear broth, but you have to bring with you a little vial or a small plastic bag containing two heaping tablespoons of fine bran (or three tablespoons of bran flakes). Dump this in your broth, and then eat it as your lunch. When your luncheon companions inquire, either answer their questions or just say it is your secret project. I have given both of these answers, depending on my mood. It is also interesting to speculate with your friends about the reaction in the kitchen, when the soup bowl returns with the residue the staff cannot identify as something they have served.

It will probably be very easy for you to keep a number of vials of bran in your desk or locker at work. Two tablespoons of fine bran or three tablespoons of bran flakes should be in each vial. When you have to go out for lunch, just grab one and stick it in your pocket, and lunch will be an easy meal to include in your diet.

Midafternoon snack. Again, if you can do without it, do so. If you cannot, follow the instructions for the midmorning snack. You may have any of the beverages listed under lunch at any time.

Dinner. Here is where you may have a ball. You may have as much as you desire, but keep in mind that this is not a contest to see how much you can eat. If you follow my recommendations, the high-fiber content of your food will make your consumption self-limiting. Unless you have a rare, special reason not to do this, you should begin dinner with bran in a broth, wait ten minutes and drink an eight-ounce glass of water or other beverage during that time.

The main-course reducing recipes listed in Chapter 11 take advantage of the many truly good low-calorie foods available. They are weighted heavily in the direction of vegetables and fruits, as your own food consumption should be. Use fish, chicken, and turkey freely, but deemphasize other meats because of their high calorie content. If this seems contrary to a previous diet that you've used, accept it nonetheless, because it is true. Red meat contains 100 calories per ounce, primarily because of its fat content. Also use condiments, spices, and sauces freely, or anything else that will make each meal more interesting and good tasting.

There is one basic combination of foods that I could eat seven nights a week and not become bored. The secret is in the variations, because I can flavor it many different ways and produce more than seven different dishes. These dishes start with mushrooms, onions, and farmer cheese. The flavor of this basic combination can be varied by using green peppers, celery, carrots, or a host of other ingredients. Meat, fish, or turkey may be added, but they are not absolutely necessary.

Spices, sauces, and seasonings are the magic wand by which these ingredients become tasty dishes. For example, by adding a little tomato paste, an eighth of a pound of meat per person, Italian herb seasoning, garlic, etc., you can make an Italian dish. On another night chicken can be added, even out of a can, and flavored with a chicken bouillon cube. Some Chinese vegetables and soy sauce can be used to produce a Chinese dish, or you can add beef or chicken and lots of paprika to produce a Hungarian-style dish. If you want a seafood night, cook the dish with fish, shrimp, or scallops, and season it with lemon juice and imitation butter flavoring.

I certainly don't want to suggest that the variations on this one dish are all that you may have for dinner. I use this example only as a model for the style of cooking that you should be doing, a style that mixes vegetables, sauces, and combinations of ingredients.

In case you're wondering if I have omitted something from

the above recipes, you are right. Each of these dishes should contain some bran, and this style of cooking is recommended because it makes the bran invisible. The bran will become lost in these dishes, and you will not taste it. At most, it will thicken the sauce; to compensate, add a little extra water.

How much bran should you use? Since each person must have a minimum of three tablespoons at dinner, you may add this amount for each portion cooked, or you may add less but supply the remaining bran in the cup of soup eaten as the first course. I recommend the two-course approach because you will feel full either way, but your body will receive fewer calories if you eat the soup.

In Chapter 11 you will find other recipes for reducing dinners. Don't forget that three tablespoons of bran are only a minimum, and by adding it in both soup and other dishes, you can have four or five tablespoons of bran with your meal.

There are also various flavorings that add a delicious new dimension to your cooking. I have previously mentioned Marmite. It is a flavoring that I first discovered in England, but is also manufactured in Canada and sold in the United States in the gourmet section of the supermarket. It comes in a small jar and has the consistency of thick, dark molasses, though it softens with heat. It has a very strong flavor of meat, but it is actually a yeast extract. In tiny amounts it adds a delicious meaty flavor to dishes. If you decide to taste it right out of the jar, use no more than a speck because it is so concentrated that it does not taste good straight. Recently, I discovered two other brands that appear to be similar or identical flavorings. These are usually available only in health-food stores and are called Vegex and Savorex.

Another flavoring that I find extremely useful is imitation butter flavoring, which is a liquid that comes in a small bottle, or imitation butter-flavored salt. Both of them are found in the spice section of the supermarket. They do an excellent job of improving certain dishes, and they are referred to in the recipe section.

Garlic flavors, such as garlic powder, garlic salt, or garlic juice can help a dish tremendously, if you like this flavor. Worcestershire sauce is fine. Even the thicker steak sauces or barbecue sauces can be used, but since these have some calories, be careful about the quantity. I encourage you to be inventive and clever, and if you come up with a dish or a style of cooking that is truly stupendous, write me about it and I'll pass it on to others. My address is listed in Chapter 9.

Beverages, again, are coffee and tea (with artificial sweetener if you want it), water, or diet sodas.

Dessert may consist of fresh fruit or unsweetened canned fruit. Incidentally, it should be noted that fruit juices are not permitted at all on the reducing diet. They are in the category of refined carbohydrates. They are generally the sugar portion of the fruit stripped of its fiber, and only provide you naked calories.

Late-night snack. You may have an apple, a pear, a couple of plums, an orange, or a comparable serving of virtually any fruit. Always eat the skin of the fruit, except when it is a rind, such as on an orange or grapefruit. I suggest that on the reducing diet you exclude such extremely high-calorie fruits as avocados and mangoes.

A very good way of judging quickly the value of any snack food, such as the fruit, is by the carbohydrate-fiber ratio. You may have as a snack any fruit with a C/F less than 25. These C/F ratios are found alphabetically in the table in Chapter 12.

THE C/F CEILING

I have set a C/F of 25 as the maximum allowable on The High-Fiber Reducing Diet. But I'm not going to tell you that this is a final limit. Like Wilbur and Orville Wright who flew above the chains of gravity, you can rise beyond this limit and eat a wider variety of foods, as long as you use the right techniques for breaking through the C/F ceiling of 25.

If you modify the foods that are over 25 by adding bran to them, you can eat them while you are on the reducing diet. Usually one or two teaspoons of bran per serving per person is sufficient.

You are only permitted to modify and eat foods that are under 100 on the C/F tables. Foods over 100 are forbidden. Add one heaping teaspoon of bran to any food with a C/F up to 60, and two heaping teaspoons to foods between 60 and 100.

Also, you are not allowed to eat a food with a C/F higher than 25 by saying that instead of adding bran to it, you'll eat the bran separately, in something else. That defeats your purpose.

Medical studies show that the food you eat is not churned into a homogeneous mass in your stomach. Each food tends to remain in separate layers, in the order it was eaten. The only way to cover the naked calories in a food with a C/F over 25 is for every mouthful of it to contain bran. Every individual naked calorie must be covered, not the meal as a whole, so each serving of a food over a C/F of 25 must contain bran or you cannot eat it.

FOLLOW THE WEIGHT-LOSS ROAD

So that you can have a complete checklist to review from time to time, the following points cover almost everything you need to know about the reducing diet. Be sure to read them frequently when you begin using this diet.

1. I cannot know what individual medical problems each of you may have. Consult your doctor before embarking on this or any other weight-reduction program. Since this program is nutritionally sound, even if your doctor is not aware of the current findings on fiber, there should be no general objection. If he or she has any questions, I would be pleased to respond. My address for correspondence is given in Chapter 9.

2. Add at least 7 grams of fiber daily in the form of unprocessed bran. Nine heaping tablespoons of bran flakes will provide the 7 grams of fiber. You can make fine-ground bran yourself (see Appendix D). Six heaping tablespoons of fine bran will provide the proper daily amount.

3. The amounts of fiber specified are minimums. Actually, the more the better.

4. Take one third of the bran with each meal. This means three heaping tablespoons of bran flakes added to each meal, or, if fine bran is used, two heaping tablespoons.

5. You are not allowed to eat refined sugar of any kind. This includes white sugar, brown sugar, "raw" sugar, honey, or molasses. The use of artificial sweeteners is permitted as a substitute for sugar.

6. The only flour that may be used is whole wheat flour, and this must be in limited amounts. See Chapter 11 for recipes.

7. Regardless of how much fluid you drink with each meal (and there is no limitation on fluid), drink one full eight-ounce glass of water about fifteen minutes after every meal. This even applies to dinner where you have already had a glass of water earlier. A diet soda or a cup of tea or coffee can substitute.

8. As I said in Chapter 6, the use of bran must be started slowly and increased gradually over a two-week period. Under no circumstances should you begin by adding 7 extra grams of fiber daily. During the first two weeks, your weight-loss results will be inadequate, but after a lifetime of eating low-fiber foods, you cannot plunge indiscriminately in the opposite direction. Use the following schedule to accustom yourself to this new diet:

· for the first three days use one heaping teaspoon of bran three times a day

· on the fourth, fifth, and sixth days use two heaping teaspoons of bran three times a day

· on the seventh, eighth, and ninth days use one heaping tablespoon of bran three times a day

· on the tenth, eleventh, and twelfth days use two heaping tablespoons of bran three times a day

· then, on the thirteenth or fourteenth day, begin using three tablespoons of bran three times a day

During this introductory period, make the following adjustments in your breakfast, lunch, and dinner:

Breakfast: Use larger amounts of the unsweetened granola cereal, gradually reducing the number of tablespoons of cereal as you increase the bran until the final proportions are reached by the fourteenth day.

Lunch: Eat a sandwich on one slice of whole wheat bread with your soup (or on two slices of thinly sliced whole wheat bread), gradually increasing the bran in the soup according to the schedule.

Dinner: Eat the meals suggested in the reducing diet, gradually increasing the amount of bran to three heaping tablespoons.

9.   Use flavorings, spices, and sauces freely to produce interesting variations in your meals. Steak and barbecue sauces containing some calories can be used, but in reasonable quantities.

10.   Take one ordinary multiple-vitamin tablet daily. It is not necessary to take a high-potency therapeutic vitamin.

11.   Most dishes will require bran to be mixed into them, because on The High-Fiber Reducing Diet each food eaten must have a C/F of less than 25. Taking the bran in broth before the meal does *not* satisfy the requirement if the individual foods eaten during the meal have a C/F ratio above 25. Then, you must add bran to each food.

12.   Chicken or turkey may be eaten freely if the skin is removed.

13.   You may have beef one or two times daily, if you wish, but it should be very lean and no more than one eighth of a pound per serving. Pork, pork products, or prepared luncheon meats should not be eaten because of their high fat and calorie content.

14. You should have fish at least twice a week.

15. You should have one serving of liver every week.

16. You must limit the use of fats and oils, and they should not be used for cooking.

17. You may have a salad with your main meal, if you wish, but it must have a C/F less than 25 (see Chapter 11). You may use only bottled dietetic dressings or those in the recipe section.

18. If you wish to have milk, use only skim milk.

19. During the reducing diet phase there should be absolutely no deviations from this diet.

20. Once you have achieved your desired weight, go directly to The Weight-Maintenance Diet.

The High-Fiber Reducing Diet combines the best of two medical worlds. On the one hand, it is a low-calorie diet, which is the recognized medical procedure for weight loss. On the other hand, it is a high-fiber diet, which provides you with a great deal of the bulk you need and satisfies your hunger.

Of course, I recommend plenty of fluids and adequate exercise to you. I make this recommendation to all my patients. Unless you are one of the few people who cannot exercise because of a medical problem, you have no excuse!

When you combine all the suggestions I recommend—high fiber for plenty of food to eat, low-calorie intake, vitamins, plenty of fluids, adequate exercise—and top them off with improved health, you've got the winning reducing diet for which I've searched for seventeen years. Now get out there and take advantage of it! It'll be the best move you ever made!

CHAPTER 9

THE NATIONAL HEALTH PROGRAM

The National Health Program offered in this chapter shows that a great deal can be done to try to reduce and perhaps eradicate both obesity and the Naked Calorie Disease throughout the United States. In a few moments you will see how this health improvement can be achieved, but first I must discuss the most important participant in every effort to gain better health—you.

Here's what I want you to do. Empty your sugar bowl of refined sugar; if you still feel you require the sweetness, fill it with granulated artificial sweetener. Next, raid the pantry and freezer and throw out all your cakes and cookies. While you're cleaning your freezer, don't forget to throw out the ice cream. If you must eat some ice cream, use the low-calorie variety. Diet soft drinks should be used instead of the heavily sugared kind. Also, switch your family to whole wheat bread instead of white bread. If you do all this and add fiber to your diet, you will be well on the way to better nutrition and health. As the Greeks said, "Well begun is half done."

You might think I'm a dreamer because I'm asking you to end your consumption of sweets, or switch from sugar to artificial sweeteners. The American public is known for ignoring sound advice that will improve its health. It didn't listen about cigarettes. It knows that cigarette smoking can lead to lung cancer, but more cigarettes are bought than ever.

I'm not a dreamer. As the evidence shows, the controversy over cigarette smoking and lung cancer is a tempest in a teapot compared to the Naked Calorie Disease. "Smoking causes lung cancer" sounds serious because lung cancer kills more people than any other form of cancer. But this smoking and lung cancer controversy is no more important than any one single facet of the complex epidemic caused by the Naked Calorie Disease. Don't forget these facts:

· Coronary disease kills twice as many people each year as all forms of cancer combined, and coronary artery disease, which is part of the Naked Calorie Disease, is the most common form of heart attack.

· There is also cancer of the colon. Every year this strikes more people than lung cancer, but it is not as deadly—it is only the second-biggest killer among cancers.

· Then there is diverticulitis, which strikes one American out of every three over the age of forty-five, and two out of three over the age of eighty.

· Add on polyps of the colon, which strikes one out of five adults; in this disease, up to 7 percent of all polyps eventually become cancerous.

· As if these weren't enough, there is diabetes, peptic ulcer, gallstones, appendicitis, tooth decay, varicose veins, and God knows what else. These diseases, taken together, constitute a greater problem than lung cancer.

· But I haven't finished, because there is also obesity, which strikes approximately one out of every two Americans. Obesity doesn't even have an incubation period; it can begin in infancy. The excess weight carried by over 100 million Americans is vivid proof that every one of us suffers a constant attack from the Naked Calorie Disease. The proof of this appears undeniable. Every time you look in the mirror and see excess pounds on your body, you are also seeing that the Naked Calorie Disease has already reached into your home. After reading this book, you will know how to fight back against these diseases and help prevent them from striking you or your family.

Your predicament doesn't even compare to smoking ciga-rettes. Most people still smoke because lung cancer seems remote. They think it will not arrive until they reach a vague and indefinable future date. But the Naked Calorie Disease could al-ready be visibly affecting your body, and your body may have already visibly degenerated. You can look at your present phys-ical condition and imagine the impact this disease has already had, and the more serious consequences that may come closer each and every day you fail to act.

I wonder how many of you really see the full magnitude of this epidemic on the health of our society, which includes you and your family. I have thought about it a great deal, and it's frightening. It's doubly frightening to me, because I'm a doctor, and I know every limitation doctors face when they try to cure each of these diseases. These are *degenerative* diseases. Once you contract any one of them you have crossed an invisible line—and there is almost no hope that you can get back to the other side of the line, no matter how faithfully you follow your doctor's instructions. When they strike suddenly, you discover that you are snowballing down a mountainside, your precious health inexorably failing you, and you are unable to stop your-self from falling all the way to the bottom.

I know that your life means a lot to you. I have tried to put myself behind your eyes and feel inside me what you might ex-perience when you commit yourself to better health and this diet: "This is it. At this moment I don't have these ailments, and I don't want to get them. True, I'm overweight, but at last I know how to get rid of my excess weight forever. True, I've got a mouth full of silver, and my body isn't what it once was—but I know it could be in much better condition again." Then you might pause, bite your lower lip and stare into space as you come to a deeper realization. "He's right. In other families (and perhaps in my own) I've seen loved ones die of heart attacks, and I've observed the misery of diabetes and cancer. I care too much for myself and my family to fall apart and become a bur-den on those whom I love. Thank God there's hope to regain better health and escape all these diseases! Today I start fresh!''

Even though most of you have made this commitment, a few may still be looking for an easier way out. These few may be saying to themselves, ''This book is undoubtedly correct, but there are other ways of losing weight, and they work too. I've lost weight on fourteen different occasions, using fourteen different methods. Even if Dr. Siegal is correct, there are other diets that are more appealing. Maybe I'll try the whipped cream diet next.''

Let's take a look at some of these other ways to lose weight. Have you tried the doctor's diet that advocates the use of only protein foods and is completely devoid of fats and carbohydrates? You know the one. It's the diet without any fiber in it whatsoever, where you have to drink gallons of water or else your stool becomes so hard you may never have another bowel movement. It isn't important that it produces ketosis, which can be damaging to the kidneys. Some people use it anyway.

Perhaps you'd like to develop your ketosis another way, and you follow that other doctor's diet. He lets you eat lots of meat and fat, but keeps the carbohydrates to a minimum. He even lets you play doctor and check your own urine, to see how bad the ketosis has become.

Then there is the diet that comes in a can. You don't even need a kitchen. All you have to do is open four cans a day, and drink down the milkshake. That should be easy to do for a few months. Besides, you can always take laxatives.

What about those shots you've been hearing about, the ones that come from the urine of pregnant women? That shouldn't be hard to do, especially with that five-hundred-calorie-a-day diet that goes with it. Maybe you could get the whole five hundred calories at one time by having a hot fudge sundae once a day?

Have you tried behavior modification? Have you tried hypnosis? Have you tried lecithin, vinegar, kelp, and vitamin B-6?

Take your pick. You can go to The Diet Control Center, The Diet Workshop, Weight Watchers, Diet Watchers, or Overeaters Anonymous.

I don't think that you can permanently solve your problem by any method that does not recognize the fiber deficiency of your present diet. The evidence presented shows that obesity is one part of a huge environmental disease, and that when the parent disease is eradicated, your obesity vanishes while your whole health picture is improved. But you don't have to listen to my recitation of the medical facts.

You can ignore me and read *Eat and Become Slim, Calories Don't Count, Eat, Drink and Get Thin,* or *The Ladies Home Journal Diet.*

If you insist, your diet can be pleasurable. You can try the Drinking Man's Diet, or the Sex Can Keep You Slim Diet.

Or you can simply buy one of the many diet programs on the market. There is the Prudent Diet, the Carbo-Cal Diet, the Boston Police Diet, the Grapefruit Diet, the New York Health Department Diet, the Zen Macrobiotic Diet, the Nova Scotia Diet, the North Pole Slenderizing Plan, the Working Man's Diet, the Nine-Day Wonder Diet, Fat-Free Forever Diet, the Natural Low-Carbo Diet, the Anti-Cellulite Diet, the Eat Sweets Diet, the Gourmet Diet, Dr. Sarley's Wine Diet, the Olympic Diet, the Organic Weighing Game, the Amazing New-You Diet, the Meat Is Enough Diet, the Beautiful People's Diet, the Lazy Lady Diet, the Computer Diet, the Candy Diet, the Ice Cream Diet, the Yogurt Diet, and the ten new diets that were published while you were reading this list.

Virtually none of these diets takes into account the body's need for a wide variety of essential nutrients. Virtually none is based on any scientific evidence whatsoever. Most important of all, virtually none has helped anybody *permanently.*

As I mentioned before, the most glaring defect of all these approaches is that they do not treat the real cause of obesity, and that's why your weight starts climbing as soon as you go off of these diets. Obesity is part of the Naked Calorie Disease, which is an environmental disease. The only successful cure for obesity is to treat the Naked Calorie Disease, and that means adding fiber and eliminating refined carbohydrates. You cannot solve obesity merely by following one diet program or another temporarily. These are sweeping you rapidly down river to a cliff where you will be washed over a towering waterfall. If you look closely at this waterfall, you will see that it is made of millions of human bodies instead of water. Amazingly enough, most of those bodies have used one popular diet or another, but they never lost their excess weight permanently.

The federal government has not been too helpful in solving our society's nutritional problems, but in some ways it has made an honest effort. The Food and Drug Administration tries, and in many ways it does protect our health. At times it becomes overprotective or fails to act, and there is an outcry of indignation, but in general it makes an honest attempt. The regulators and legislative bodies are torn between whom they should believe, with forward-looking medical researchers on one side and pressure from the giant food interests with their own staffs of product designers on the other. In spite of all government efforts, consumer education in the nutritional field has failed, and the public is baffled by huge food-advertising campaigns while only occasional newspaper and magazine stories carry opposing reports from medical authorities. After all, how constant a stream of these contradictory stories can TV, magazines, and newspapers provide? A major part of their advertising revenues comes from the food manufacturers.

A war on the naked calorie is a way around all this—it is a war that can build a solid bridge between all sides—government, industry, and consumer—and provide better health for the public. In fact, this is one war where nobody loses his or her life, but one in which you win your life. If we lose this war we lose our health, our loved ones, and our money. If we win, we will have defeated one of the biggest and most destructive enemies our country has ever faced.

TOGETHER WE CAN WIN!

My best medical opinion is that the first thing you should do is help yourself. Take off that excess weight and proceed with The Weight-Maintenance Diet. If you are smart you will do this now—and you will probably be in time to prevent the naked calorie from causing you the worst harm. If you are over the age of forty, it may have already taken quite a toll on your health, but you can at least prevent further damage. After you have made your inner commitment and taken your first steps toward saving yourself, you may want to turn your attention to the health of our society.

This is like any other war, and it cannot be fought without an army. A strong organization, with devoted workers, is needed. I envision a new national health foundation that is built on a solid base of medical and nonmedical personnel *who care.*

The March of Dimes successfully conquered polio. The American Cancer Society supports a great number of research projects that study cancer. There are many other medical foundations, each with its own disease, such as cystic fibrosis and multiple sclerosis. The organization I envision would be a new health foundation—but it would be different. Since it already knows how to prevent the diseases it must fight, its goal would be the elimination of the huge epidemic caused by the Naked Calorie Disease.

I see the goal of this foundation as the improvement of the eating habits and therefore the health of the American people—through public education by a national health campaign, through working with the food industry to supply additional high-fiber products, and through enlistment of our legislators to protect us with laws.

· The organization's Board of Directors should represent as wide a public as possible.
· It should include members from publishing and other communications media.

· There should be representatives from a variety of social, ethnic, and economic groups.

· There would be a continuing invitation offered to food manufacturers and restauranteurs, so industry may provide products that satisfy evolving public and market demand. In this way industry may become a partner in providing better health, instead of a distant adversary.

· Doctors, nutritionists, and a variety of specialists, such as cancer and heart disease researchers, should join this growing national partnership, and,

· At all times, the organization's ear should be turned toward the food and health concerns voiced by the general public, and the organization's energies should be aimed toward helping the public meet its good eating needs.

There could be local branches all over the country that would work to advance high-fiber nutrition at the grass-roots level. In the same way that "stop smoking" centers and programs are available in every community, high-fiber nutrition centers can also spring up and offer programs that have received the organization's seal of approval.

I foresee a vast membership drive for wide participation, with nominal membership fees paying the expenses of the foundation's campaigns and guarantees that no individual would profit from the organization.

These nominal membership dues would support a number of important programs. There would be periodic "fiber" conferences or conventions, at which medical authorities would present the latest advances. These conferences would receive sufficient press coverage to inform the general public of the latest findings.

A permanent foundation staff would prepare and publish a "working program" that specifies changes the food manufacturers should make in each kind of product. These changes would primarily be to include fiber in foods, to eliminate sugar, and to substitute whole wheat flour for white flour. This staff would also monitor new food products entering the market and try to persuade their manufacturers to use fiber and artificial sweeteners.

The foundation might also take its message to Washington, bringing its case before the legislative committees of both houses of Congress and into the conference rooms of the Food and Drug Administration.

It would work in harmony with the Food and Drug Administration, medical associations, food manufacturing associations, and restaurant associations.

There might be a campaign in many cities to enlist participation by local restaurants and by food franchise chains that span the continent. They could each carry some fiber-rich choices on their menus. The foundation staff would make it easy for them by providing suggestions and recipes tailored to different kinds of restaurants serving different varieties of foods. Participating restaurants could be identified by some decal or symbol at the door, which they could also use in their advertising.

Millions of people eat "institutional food" in corporate cafeterias, hospitals, nursing homes, colleges, public schools, etc. There might also be a campaign to provide this institutional-food industry with recipes and fiber-addition suggestions.

The foundation could also purchase a small number of shares of stock in many of the large food corporations and attempt to communicate its position through shareholders' referendums.

Citizens who join this national health campaign might receive a regular publication that would include new research information, tasty high-fiber recipes, recommendations for weight loss and better health, as well as warnings against certain types of fad diets.

The foundation would need workers or "soldiers" in many areas of expertise. It would stimulate and help financially support research projects on the use of fiber in the American diet, as well as the very important, almost untouched field of the use of fiber in infant nutrition. Hopefully, many members of this organization would volunteer for large-scale statistical research on the lowered disease rates of various age groups utilizing high-fiber diets.

The members could also carry out letter-writing campaigns to Washington and to the food industry, and this could have a powerful impact.

This would be a dedicated and responsible foundation whose every step is positive, never negative, where no manufacturer or restaurant is singled out and condemned for the products it produces, but where each is encouraged by aggressive and honest public action to provide alternatives in the form of new and healthier foods and restaurant dishes.

If this new health campaign is truly successful, many present products would have fiber added to them, and their sugar content would be eliminated or replaced by other kinds of sweeteners. In essence, these would be new products. They would bear the same names we see in our supermarkets today and come in the same packages—yet they would be much healthier for us to eat. Our society would owe these manufacturers and restaurants a large debt of gratitude.

If you would like to be part of this nonviolent, highly beneficial war, please drop me a line. A postcard with your name and address will do. Address it to: Dr. Sanford Siegal, Post Office Box 480870, Miami, Florida 33148.

We all know the tremendous impact that a well-organized disease-fighting foundation can have on public health. The March of Dimes conquered polio solely on the strength of public involvement and commitment. Government money was not spent, yet this dread disease has been defeated.

The citizens of our country have the talent, skill, and energy to successfully tackle and perhaps even eradicate the Naked Calorie Disease. Experienced public health professionals who could staff and run the foundation's national health campaign are available. The doctors, lawyers, concerned citizens, journalists, fund-raisers, and the other specialized talents needed locally are present in every city and town in our country. It is my firm belief that once this new national health foundation is established, it will generate broad public support that will sustain an active program. Our nation *can* conquer the Naked Calorie Disease. Americans can enjoy a great improvement in their health, in addition to the virtual elimination of obesity from our society. Is this a victory worth winning? You bet it is! It's a war on disease we can win—and we should begin today!

CHAPTER 10

RULES TO REMEMBER

This chapter is included to give you a quick summary of the basic rules for my two diets, which were explained fully in Chapters 7 and 8. At first you should refer back to these chapters frequently to be sure that you are still on the right track. Afterward, check these rules or the specific chapters if you have a question.

The Weight-Maintenance Diet

1. See your doctor and tell him or her about this diet. You should have an examination before you start any diet.
2. Begin the program using the two-week introductory period described in Chapter 6.
3. Add nine heaping tablespoons of bran to your daily diet, three to each meal.
4. Eat no refined sugar or brown sugar. As for honey or molasses, see Chapter 7.
5. Eat no refined flour, only whole wheat flour.
6. Consult the C/F tables about any food of which you are not sure.
7. Eat only foods with a C/F below 100, or those with a B rating that you have supplemented with bran (see Chapter 12).
8. Drink fluids at any time, but you must have a glass of

water or other beverage fifteen minutes after each meal. Also drink a glass of water or other beverage at bedtime.

9. Take one multiple-vitamin capsule daily.

10. Get sufficient exercise.

The High-Fiber Reducing Diet

1. See your doctor and tell him or her about this diet. You should have an examination before you start any diet.

2. Begin by following the rules for the two-week introductory period described in Chapter 6.

3. Add nine heaping tablespoons of bran to your daily diet, three to each meal.

4. Eat no refined sugar, brown sugar, honey, or molasses.

5. Eat no refined flour, only whole wheat flour.

6. Begin dinner with the bran-broth mixture, and then wait ten minutes before eating the remainder of the meal. While you wait drink an eight-ounce glass of water.

7. Consult the C/F tables about any food of which you are not sure.

8. Eat only foods with a C/F below 25, or foods with an S rating that you have supplemented with bran. Foods with a T rating may be eaten cautiously (see Chapter 12).

9. In addition to other fluids, drink one glass of water with dinner (see rule 6), one glass after each of the three meals, and one at bedtime.

10. Take one multiple-vitamin capsule daily.

11. Get sufficient exercise.

12. When you have achieved your desired weight, proceed directly to The Weight-Maintenance Diet.

RECIPES

High-fiber cooking. The recipes presented in this chapter are in conventional form, but they are not conventional. In fact, they introduce you to a new style of cooking, high-fiber cooking "American style," and this has never existed before. Remember that you don't have to follow these recipes exactly. They are provided to guide you safely into this new world of high-fiber cooking.

The problem with developing this new style of cooking is obvious. There isn't any information available on this subject anywhere. High-fiber cooking had to be created from the ground up. Make no mistake about it: I have been extremely careful in doing this. Every one of these recipes has been tested, and all of them taste fine.

Use your judgment. Your cooking preferences may be different from mine. Since I am an avid amateur cook, I know that even when I follow a recipe for the first time, I make my own personal variations. At times the changes are made almost automatically, since I find it impossible not to add or subtract from the ingredients according to my own likes and dislikes. I expect most of you to do the same, adding a little more of this or a little less of that, including brand-new ingredients or deleting others. This will be true with the spices and seasonings. Some of these recipes are well seasoned, but if you like less seasoning in your food, you can either reduce their amounts or delete them altogether. Use your judgment.

Go ahead and use your personal preferences, but abide by the rules. What are these rules? There are two areas of cooking where I have made changes—adding fiber and substituting a sweetener for sugar. Each of these changes has its own table right here, in the front of the recipe section, to ease your way.

RULE #1: ADD FIBER

The first change is to be sure you add fiber to each dish that contains carbohydrate, meaning generally those foods that come from the ground. Each mouthful of carbohydrate must have its fiber, so that you don't receive any naked calories.

In the recipes the teaspoons and tablespoons of bran are always *heaping.* You can add more than this suggested amount, according to your taste.

There are two kinds of bran you can use. Each has a table of its own. The first is the regular, unprocessed miller's bran that is sold in all health-food stores. It is in the form of very small flakes. The second is fine bran, which you make at home by grinding the regular bran in an inexpensive electric grinder. (A blender won't work.) For questions on how to make fine bran, see Appendix D, which lists the different grinders you may buy and use.

Many of the recipes suggest fine bran. If you do not have a grinder, you can also use the following two tables to judge how much bran to substitute for the fine bran.

Just how much fiber are you actually getting? The following two tables provide the answer. The first table is for regular bran and the second is for fine bran. Refer to these tables whenever you have to decide the amount of fiber that you need to add to your own recipes, or even to each meal.

FIBER CONTAINED IN VARIOUS MEASURES OF BRAN

Amount of Bran	Amount of Fiber (gms)	Amount of Fiber Per Serving (gms)					
		1	2	3	4	5	6
1 heaping tsp.	0.28	0.28	0.14	0.09	0.07	0.06	.0.05
1 heaping tbsp.	0.80	0.80	0.40	0.27	0.20	0.16	0.13
2 heaping tbsp.	1.60	1.60	0.80	0.53	0.40	0.32	0.27
3 heaping tbsp.	2.40	2.40	1.20	0.80	0.60	0.48	0.40
1 level cup	5.60	5.60	2.80	1.90	1.40	1.10	0.93

FIBER CONTAINED IN VARIOUS MEASURES OF FINE BRAN

Amount of Fine Bran	Amount of Fiber (gms)	Amount of Fiber Per Serving (gms)					
		1	2	3	4	5	6
1 heaping tsp.	0.55	0.55	0.28	0.18	0.14	0.11	0.09
1 heaping tbsp.	1.10	1.10	0.55	0.36	0.28	0.22	0.18
2 heaping tbsp.	2.20	2.20	1.10	0.73	0.55	0.44	0.37
3 heaping tbsp.	3.20	3.20	1.60	1.10	0.80	0.64	0.53
1 level cup	7.10	7.10	3.60	2.40	1.80	1.40	1.20

RULE #2: SUBSTITUTE A SWEETENER FOR SUGAR

The second change in your cooking habits is to substitute a dietetic sweetener for sugar. You shouldn't even have sugar in the house. You, your family, and your guests will be better off if you substitute other sweeteners for sugar.

There are a number of dietetic sweeteners available. I have listed most of them in alphabetical order in the following table, where you will find the quantity of each of them to use for an equivalent amount of sugar. This table will come in handy for recipes that call for sweetening, as I have listed the sweetening ingredients in the following way:

dietetic sweetener = 3 teaspoons sugar

When you see this in a recipe, simply look at the following chart. Find the name of your brand of sweetener, and read across the line to see how much of it to use. After the first two or three recipes, you will probably begin to remember how much of your brand of sweetener you need to use for an equivalent amount of sugar. Or you may wish to write the equivalent amount on the top of your box of sweetener, so it is immediately available.

TABLE OF SWEETENING EQUIVALENTS

Name	Form	Equivalent to 1 tsp. Sugar	Equivalent to 2 tsp. Sugar	Equivalent to 1 cup Sugar
Sakrin	Liquid	2 drops		
Sprinkle Sweet	Granulated	1 tsp.		1 cup
Sucaryl	Granulated	1 tsp.		1 cup
Sucaryl	Liquid	1/8 tsp.		
Sucaryl	Tablets	1 tablet		
Sugar Twin	Granulated	1 tsp.		1 cup
Sugar Twin Brown	Granulated	1 tsp. (brown sugar)		
Sugar Twin	Packets		1 packet	
Sug'r Like	Granulated	1 tsp.		1 cup
Superose	Liquid	4 drops		1 tbsp.
Sweeta	Liquid	2 drops		
Sweeta	Tablets	1 tablet		
Sweet 'n Low	Granulated	1/10 tsp.*		4 tsp.
Sweet 'n Low	Packets		1 packet	
Sweet ★ 10	Liquid	10 drops		2 tbsp.
Weight Watchers	Granulated	1 tsp.		1 cup
Weight Watchers	Packets		1 packet	
Neeta-Sweet	Packets		1 packet	
Neeta-Sweet (1/2 grain)	Tablets		1 tablet	

* 1/10 tsp. measuring spoon enclosed in package.

This table includes most of the sweeteners that are commonly available. It is not meant to list every sweetening product on the market.

In addition, there are many brands of saccharin tablets on the market. They generally come in 3 strengths, ¼ grain, ½ grain, and 1 grain. Here are their approximate sugar-sweetness equivalents:

¼ grain tablets = 1 tsp.
½ grain tablets = 2 tsp.
1 grain tablets = 4 tsp.

SERVING SIZE

All the recipes included here are designed to give two ample servings unless otherwise indicated. The recipes can be cut in half for one person, or doubled for four people, or easily adjusted for three by adding half again to each quantity. The fiber content of each recipe, per serving, is given so that you can keep a running total for the day. Remember, you need 10 to 12 grams of fiber daily, and it should be distributed fairly equally among all three meals.

AN EXTRA HINT FOR DIETERS

The carbohydrate-fiber ratio of each recipe is also given. Those of you who are reducing are encouraged to make the broadest use of those ingredients with the lowest C/F. Take time to look through the C/F tables in Chapter 12. You will discover that you can use many low C/F foods in imaginative combinations with a variety of seasonings, and thus produce a much greater selection of menus than is suggested by the recipes in this chapter. Dieters should also remember that the suggested quantities of bran are only minimums, and they can add more.

RATING THE RECIPES

USE THIS RATING SYSTEM. IT IS VERY IMPORTANT. This rating system is used in both this recipe chapter and, in expanded form, in the C/F tables. It tells you whether a recipe is recommended for The High-Fiber Reducing Diet or whether it is acceptable only on The Weight-Maintenance Diet. It works like this:

Rating	Explanation
M	Acceptable on The Weight-Maintenance Diet
R	Acceptable on The High-Fiber Reducing Diet

The tables in Chapter 12 use five other categories, N, S, T, X, and Y. There isn't any need for these categories in the recipes, so they appear and are explained only in Chapter 12.

A FINAL REMINDER

One last reminder before I turn you loose and give you free rein in this "new world" of high-fiber cooking: you must introduce fiber to your diet gradually over a two-week period. The schedule to follow is covered in Chapters 6 and 8. If you introduce fiber to your diet gradually, you will feel better and you will be much more successful.

BREAKFAST

FLASHY ONION 'N EGGS

Fiber per serving	**0.6**	*1 small onion diced*
C/F	**8.8**	*12 tablespoons Second Nature =*
Rating	**M, R**	*4 eggs*
		⅛ teaspoon salt
		¼ cup cottage cheese
		2 heaping teaspoons bran

Heat a no-stick frying pan sprayed with vegetable coating. Sautée onions until transparent. In a mixing bowl, beat the rest of the ingredients together. Add the mixture to the onions and scramble. Cook over medium heat until eggs are done.

FRENCH TOAST

Fiber per serving	0.7	6 tablespoons Second Nature
C/F	17.0	(R) =2 eggs (M)
Rating	M, R	dietetic sweetener =4 teaspoons sugar
		2 teaspoons cinnamon
		1 heaping teaspoon fine bran
		2 slices whole wheat bread

Combine in mixing bowl the Second Nature, sweetener, cinnamon, and bran. Mix well until all ingredients are combined. Soak bread in mixture until moist. Heat a no-stick frying pan until hot. Add the moistened bread and cook until browned. Turn toast over and brown other side.

Instead of pan frying, bread can also be broiled or baked on aluminum foil. Broil for approximately 3 minutes on each side. Bake for approximately 5 to 6 minutes on each side, or until toast is browned.

JELLY ROLL PANCAKES

Fiber per serving	1.4	½ cup whole wheat flour
C/F	20.0	½ cup skim milk
Rating	M, R	3 tablespoons Second Nature (R) =1 egg (M)
		1 heaping tablespoon fine bran pinch of salt
		2 tablespoons dietetic jelly dietetic sweetener, to taste

In a mixing bowl combine flour and milk, and stir until very smooth. Add the Second Nature, bran, and salt. Mix very well. Spray vegetable coating on a small no-stick frying pan. Heat until pan is hot. Add ⅓ cup of batter to the pan. Tilt pan and spread batter evenly over entire pan. Cook over low heat until golden brown. Turn over, using a spatula, and brown other side. Place pancake on serving platter, and repeat until all the pancakes are cooked. Then spread a teaspoon of jelly and sprinkle some dietetic sweetener over each cooked pancake. Roll the pancake in a jelly-roll form, and serve piping hot.

WHOLE WHEAT HOT CAKES

Fiber per serving	**1.3**	*½ cup skim milk*
C/F	**19.0**	*3 tablespoons Second Nature*
Rating	**M, R**	*(R) =1 egg (M)*
		½ cup whole wheat flour
		1 heaping tablespoon fine bran
		⅛ teaspoon salt

In a mixing bowl combine and mix milk with Second Nature. Add whole wheat flour, bran, and salt. Mix thoroughly until well blended. Spray a frying pan with no-stick vegetable coating and heat pan. Place 1 tablespoon batter into hot pan and cook for about 1 to 2 minutes on each side. Repeat. Serve hot with dietetic jelly or syrup (see p. 230).

WHOLE WHEAT HOT CAKES
WITH ORANGE PIECES

Fiber per serving	**1.5**	*½ cup skim milk*
C/F	**20.0**	*3 tablespoons Second Nature*
Rating	**M, R**	*(R) = 1 egg (M)*

½ cup whole wheat flour
1 heaping tablespoon fine bran
⅛ teaspoon salt
¼ large fresh orange, cut in very
small pieces

In a mixing bowl combine milk and Second Nature. Mix well. Add whole wheat flour, bran, salt, and orange pieces. Mix thoroughly until all ingredients are well blended. In a no-stick frying pan sprayed with vegetable coating heat until pan is very hot. Place 1 tablespoon batter in hot pan and cook for about 1 to 2 minutes on each side. Repeat. Serve hot with dietetic jelly or syrup (see p. 230).

To make "Banana Hot Cakes" substitute three 1-inch pieces of banana, mashed well, for orange pieces.

CHEESE PANCAKES

Fiber per serving	**1.0**	6 tablespoons Second Nature
C/F	**14.0**	(R) = 2 eggs (M)
Rating	**M, R**	1 cup cottage cheese
		½ cup skim milk
		½ teaspoon salt
		1 heaping tablespoon fine bran
		2 slices whole wheat bread, made into crumbs (see p. 230)

Combine all the ingredients. Mix very well. Drop by heaping teaspoonfuls into a hot no-stick pan. Brown on both sides. Serve hot with dietetic jelly or syrup (see p. 230).

LUNCH

OPEN-
FACED REUBEN SANDWICH

Fiber per serving	**1.5**
C/F	**15.0**
Rating	**M, R**

2 slices whole wheat bread
4 ounces cooked sliced white meat turkey
½ cup sauerkraut, drained
2 slices Swiss cheese
1 heaping teaspoon fine bran
    Russian dressing (see p. 171)
½ dill pickle, finely minced

Slightly toast the bread. Top each piece of bread with turkey, sauerkraut, and slice of cheese. Sprinkle with bran. Spread with Russian dressing. Put under broiler until cheese melts. Garnish with pickle on each sandwich.

HOT TURKEY SANDWICH

Fiber per serving	**0.8**
C/F	**19.0**
Rating	**M, R**

2 slices whole wheat bread
4 ounces cooked white meat turkey, sliced thin
2 slices dietetic pineapple rings, drained
1 heaping teaspoon fine bran
2 slices Swiss cheese

Preheat oven to 350°. Toast bread and put on baking sheet. Place equal amount of turkey on each slice. Place a ring of pineapple on top of turkey. Sprinkle ½ teaspoon of bran on each slice. Then top each with a slice of Swiss cheese. Bake in oven for about 3 minutes or until the cheese melts.

HOT CHEESE SANDWICH

Fiber per serving	**0.8**	
C/F	**16.0**	
Rating	**M, R**	

2 slices whole wheat bread
2 slices American cheese
½ medium tomato, cut in slices
   dash of garlic salt
1 heaping teaspoon bran
½ tablespoon sesame seeds,
   toasted

Place the pieces of bread on a no-stick cookie sheet. Put under broiler for a few minutes, until one side is browned. Turn over and on the untoasted side place American cheese and tomato slices. In a bowl combine garlic salt, bran, and toasted sesame seeds. Mix together. Then sprinkle on tomatoes. Return to broiler and broil until cheese melts.

HOT MEXICAN TACOS

Fiber per serving	**1.2**	
C/F	**14.4**	
Rating	**M, R**	

6 ounces ground beef
¼ teaspoon Marmite
1 heaping tablespoon fine bran
1½ teaspoons chili powder
2 teaspoons onion flakes
½ teaspoon salt
½ teaspoon onion powder
½ teaspoon paprika
   dash of Tabasco sauce
2 slices whole wheat bread
1 cup lettuce, shredded
½ cup cottage cheese,
   blended until consistency of
   sour cream
1 tablespoon pimiento sauce
   (see p. 228)
2 toothpicks

In a no-stick skillet, brown ground beef. Add Marmite, bran, chili powder, onion flakes, salt, onion powder, paprika, and Tabasco sauce. Mix together well. When meat is browned, remove it from pan with slotted spoon so fat is left in pan. Toast the slices of bread lightly. Spread meat mixture on half of each slice and fold bread. Spoon cottage cheese (after blending to sour cream consistency) on top of meat. Next combine shredded lettuce and pimiento sauce and divide equally over cottage cheese. Fold bread again, secure with toothpicks, and serve.

DEVILED EGGS

Fiber per serving	0.3	2 hard-boiled eggs
C/F	4.0	⅛ cup vanilla yogurt
Rating	M, R	¼ teaspoon lemon juice
		⅛ teaspoon dry mustard
		pinch of garlic powder
		pinch of minced onions
		1 heaping teaspoon fine bran
		dash of paprika

After the eggs are cooked and cooled slice them in half. Remove the yolks and put them in a mixing bowl. Mash them with all the other ingredients except the paprika. Place mixture back into egg whites, stuffing as high as possible. Place in refrigerator and chill. When ready to serve sprinkle paprika on each egg.

CHEESE AND EGG SPREAD

Fiber per serving	0.6	2 hard-boiled eggs, chopped fine
C/F	4.4	
Rating	M, R	½ cup cottage cheese
		1 tablespoon skim milk

> 1 heaping tablespoon fine bran
> 2 teaspoons prepared mustard
> 1 teaspoon dried chives,
>   chopped
> ¼ teaspoon salt
>   dash of Worcestershire sauce

Combine the eggs and all the other ingredients in a bowl. Mix well. Cover the bowl and chill in the refrigerator until ready to use. Can be used with whole wheat bread as a sandwich, on lettuce leaves for a salad, or stuffed into celery stalks for a snack.

EASY EGG SOUFFLE

Fiber per serving	2.7	
C/F	17.0	
Rating	M	

8 slices whole wheat bread, crust removed
9 tablespoons Second Nature = 3 eggs
½ cup skim milk
½ teaspoon salt
2 ounces (⅛ pound) margarine
6 ounces sharp cheddar cheese, grated
2 heaping tablespoons fine bran

Cut each piece of bread into quarters. Spoon Second Nature into a bowl and add milk. Mix together. Add salt and mix. Set aside. In a small saucepan melt the margarine. Remove from heat and set aside. Grease a small 1-quart casserole or use a no-stick baking dish equal to 1 quart. Line the bottom and sides of the casserole with the bread. Pinch the pieces together to insure their staying together. Sprinkle cheese and bran over bread. Pour egg and milk mixture over cheese and soak the bread thoroughly. Pour the melted margarine over the egg and milk. Cover casserole and place in refrigerator overnight or until ready to use. When ready to use, put casserole in pan with half an inch of water to insure that mixture doesn't burn. Bake at 400° for 1½ hours.

CRABMEAT PINEAPPLE DELUXE

Fiber per serving	**2.1**
C/F	**19.6**
Rating	**M, R**

1 fresh pineapple
3 ounces canned or frozen crabmeat
1 celery stalk, finely chopped
2 tablespoons low calorie Italian dressing
½ tablespoon cottage cheese
1 heaping tablespoon fine bran
¼ teaspoon curry powder
¼ cup chopped walnuts
dash of salt
¼ medium-sized apple, chopped

Cut pineapple in half lengthwise. Leave tops on. With a knife remove "meat" from pineapple. Drain shells by turning them upside down. Then wrap in plastic bag and place in refrigerator. Using half of pineapple "meat," combine with all other ingredients. Taste to be sure there is enough salt and curry. Place salad mixture into pineapple shell. Chill and serve.

SALADS

RUSSIAN DRESSING

Fiber per serving	**0.6**	½ cup cottage cheese
C/F	**18.0**	¼ cup water
Rating	**M, R**	¼ cup ketchup
		1 heaping teaspoon fine bran
		⅛ teaspoon garlic salt
		½ small dill pickle, minced

Put all ingredients in blender. Mix very well for about 40 seconds. Pour over salads or use on sandwiches.

SALAD DRESSING

Fiber per serving	**0.7**	1 cup cottage cheese
C/F	**12.0**	1 cup water
Rating	**M, R**	1 heaping tablespoon fine bran
		2 tablespoons chopped onion
		½ teaspoon poppy seeds (optional)
		½ teaspoon dried chives (optional)
		½ teaspoon garlic, minced
		¼ teaspoon oregano
		salt and pepper to taste

Place cottage cheese, water, and bran into blender. Mix until mixture is of sour-cream consistency. Add rest of ingredients and turn on blender for 15 seconds. If mixture becomes too thick, add a few drops of water and blend again. For extra zing add ⅓ cup ketchup. Place ketchup in the blender with all the other ingredients, and mix for 10 seconds. Use as dip for cut-up raw vegetables, cooked shrimp, and cold chicken or turkey, as well as a salad dressing.

ESCAROLE SALAD

Fiber per serving	1.6	1 medium escarole
C/F	4.4	½ clove garlic, chopped
Rating	M, R	½ teaspoon butter-flavored salt
		¼ teaspoon lemon-pepper marinade
		water to cover
		1 heaping teaspoon fine bran

Wash and pat dry escarole. Put into a medium-size saucepan. Add all the seasonings and mix. Cover with water. Boil 15 to 25 minutes, until escarole is soft. Drain and squeeze out water. Chop up. Add bran and mix well. Add more butter-flavored salt, and pepper, if necessary. Cool.

SALAD WITH BEAN SPROUTS

Fiber per serving	1.9	1 pound bean sprouts, fresh or canned (16-ounce can, drained)
C/F	7.0	1 tablespoon low-calorie Thousand Island dressing
Rating	M, R	3 small green olives, chopped
		½ teaspoon wine vinegar
		½ teaspoon lemon juice
		¼ cup soy sauce
		1 tablespoon onion, chopped
		2 tablespoons pickle, chopped
		1 medium tomato, sliced
		salt and pepper to taste
		1 heaping tablespoon fine bran

Combine all ingredients except bran in a bowl. Toss together. Sprinkle bran on and toss again. Chill and serve.

TOMATO AND ONION SALAD WITH SESAME SEEDS

Fiber per serving	1.8
C/F	9.3
Rating	M

2 medium tomatoes, thinly sliced
1 medium red (mild) onion, thinly sliced
1 tablespoon sesame seeds, toasted
seasoned salt to taste
2 tablespoons vinegar
2 tablespoons oil
1 heaping teaspoon fine bran
1 tablespoon parsley flakes
½ clove garlic, mashed

Place tomatoes and onion in a salad bowl. Add the toasted sesame seeds and seasoned salt. Add the vinegar and oil and mix well. Then add bran, parsley, and garlic. Toss and chill.

MELON AND SEAFOOD SALAD

Fiber per serving	1.1
C/F	23.0
Rating	M, R

¼ pound shrimp, cut into pieces
¼ pound crab meat, flaked well
¼ cup diet Italian salad dressing
1 cup cottage cheese
¼ teaspoon seasoned salt
½ teaspoon lime juice concentrate
1 heaping teaspoon fine bran
¼ teaspoon poppy seeds
1 medium cantaloupe
2 leaves romaine lettuce
2 wedges of lemon

Combine shrimp and crab meat in a mixing bowl. Add salad dressing and mix well. Place seafood combination, covered, into refrigerator and chill for 1 hour. In another bowl combine cottage cheese, seasoned salt, lime juice, bran, and poppy seeds. Set aside. Cut cantaloupe in half. Remove seeds. Place each half on a plate. Remove fish from refrigerator and drain all the juices from it. Place half cottage cheese mixture in each cantaloupe piece, and half of seafood mixture over the cottage cheese. Place cantaloupes on pieces of lettuce and garnish each with a lemon wedge.

SHRIMP SALAD

Fiber per serving	0.5	½ pound shrimp, cooked and
C/F	5.7	cut into bite-size pieces
Rating	M, R	1 stalk celery, diced
		1 tablespoon lemon juice
		2 tablespoons mayonnaise
		salt and pepper to taste
		1 heaping teaspoon bran
		4 lettuce leaves
		2 lemon wedges (optional)

Combine shrimp with diced celery and lemon juice. Add mayonnaise, salt and pepper, and bran. Mix together well. Place 2 lettuce leaves on each plate and spoon salad on top. Garnish each with a lemon wedge.

SOUPS

GREAT GAZPACHO SOUP

Fiber per serving	1.3	¾ cup condensed beef broth
C/F	6.9	¾ cup tomato juice
Rating	M, R	1 tablespoon lemon juice

> 1   tablespoon onion, chopped
> ½   clove garlic, cut in half
> ⅛   teaspoon hot pepper sauce
> ¼   teaspoon salt
>   dash of pepper
> 2   heaping tablespoons fine
>   bran

Combine all ingredients. Place in container with cover. Shake well. Place in refrigerator for 3 to 4 hours. Remove garlic. While this is in the refrigerator, cut and then chill

> ½   green pepper, chopped fine
> ½   cucumber, chopped
> ½   tomato, chopped

Add vegetables to chilled soup just before serving.

SOUP WITH LIVER DUMPLINGS

Fiber per serving	**0.8**	
C/F	**16.0**	
Rating	**M, R**	

> ¼   pound chicken livers, cooked
> 2   slices whole wheat bread,
>   made into crumbs (see
>   p. 230)
> ⅓   cup instant nonfat dry milk
> 6   tablespoons Second Nature
>   (R) = 2 eggs (M)
> 1   tablespoon dried parsley
>
> 1   heaping teaspoon fine bran
>   salt and pepper to taste
> 2   chicken bouillon cubes
> 3   cups water

Put cooked livers through a meat grinder. Add the bread

crumbs, milk, Second Nature, parsley, bran, and salt and pepper to meat. Mix well. In a medium size saucepan add bouillon
cubes to water. Bring to a boil and dissolve the cubes. Divide
the liver mixture into 8 dumplings or balls. Drop four at a time
into the hot bouillon. Cook about 5 minutes. Remove the four
dumplings with a slotted spoon. Place them in a soup plate.
Repeat this process with the other four dumplings. Pour equal
amounts of bouillon into each bowl, over dumplings.

MAIN COURSES

CHICKEN AND RED SAUCE

Fiber per serving	1.5	
C/F	6.6	
Rating	**M, R**	

2 whole chicken breasts,
  skinned and boned
½ teaspoon onion salt
  dash of pepper
¼ teaspoon oregano
4 ounces tomato sauce
2 tablespoons fine bran
2 ounce can mushroom pieces,
  undrained
3 ounces part skim milk
  mozzarella cheese, shredded

Preheat oven to 350°. Place the chicken in a shallow baking
dish. Sprinkle on the onion salt, pepper, and oregano. In a separate bowl combine the tomato sauce, bran, and mushrooms
with its liquid. Mix well. Pour over chicken, covering the pieces
thoroughly. Bake in heated oven uncovered for approximately
30 minutes, until the chicken is soft and tender. Remove pan
from oven and sprinkle cheese over pieces. Return to oven
again for 5 to 7 minutes, until cheese melts.

CHICKEN BURGERS

Fiber per serving	0.8
C/F	11.0
Rating	M, R

1 can (5 ounces) boned chicken in broth, or 1 cup leftover chicken meat
salt and pepper to taste
3 tablespoons Second Nature (R) = 1 egg (M)
1 heaping tablespoon fine bran
1 tablespoon onion, minced
2 tablespoons ketchup
½ teaspoon celery salt

In a bowl chop chicken until very fine. Add all the other ingredients to the chicken and mix well together. Shape mixture into four patties. Place patties on a piece of foil and bake for about 5 to 8 minutes. Turn once to brown other side.

CHICKEN BREASTS PARMIGIANA

Fiber per serving	1.2
C/F	13.0
Rating	M

¼ cup whole wheat flour
1 teaspoon oregano, chopped
1 clove garlic, finely chopped
2 heaping tablespoons bran
2 chicken breasts, skinned and boned
3 ounces mozzarella cheese, cut into thin slices

Preheat oven to 450°. In a shallow plate combine flour, oregano, garlic, and bran. Moisten chicken with water. Dip the chicken breasts into the mixture, coating both sides very well. Place the coated chicken, bottom side up, on a no-stick cookie sheet and bake for 10 minutes. Turn chicken to brown other side. After 5 minutes remove from oven, place pieces of cheese over chicken, replace in oven and wait for the cheese to melt. Remove and serve hot.

FRIED CHICKEN

Fiber per serving	2.8	1 egg, beaten
C/F	8.0	½ cup milk
Rating	M	2 heaping tablespoons whole wheat flour
		6 heaping tablespoons bran
		1 teaspoon salt
		4 chicken thighs or equivalent
		½ cup cooking oil

Mix egg and milk in a shallow bowl. Mix flour, bran, and salt in another bowl. Dip chicken pieces in liquid mixture and then coat completely with dry mixture. Fry in large skillet with oil at low to medium heat for about 30 minutes.

CHICKEN LIVERS IN SCALLION SAUCE

Fiber per serving	0.6	2 packages (8 ounces each) frozen chicken livers, defrosted
C/F	6.8	3 tablespoons vinegar
Rating	M, R	3 tablespoons soy sauce
		1 heaping teaspoon fine bran

> dietetic sweetener = 3 tea-
> spoons sugar
> 1 cup chicken bouillon
> ½ cup scallions, chopped in
>   small pieces

Wipe defrosted livers dry. In a bowl combine vinegar, soy sauce, bran, sweetener, and bouillon. Put livers in a shallow baking pan. Pour about half the liquid mixture over the livers. Let stand for 15 minutes. Add scallions to other half of the liquid mixture still in the mixing bowl and set aside. Broil the livers until done, about 10 minutes. Remove from baking pan and put livers in a serving platter. Heat reserved scallion mixture and pour over livers in serving platter.

CHICKEN LIVERS ITALIANO

Fiber per serving	4.5	
C/F	7.8	
Rating	M, R	

½ pound frozen chicken livers, defrosted
5 heaping tablespoons fine bran
½ teaspoon oregano
½ teaspoon garlic, minced
   salt and pepper to taste
1 can (8 ounce) tomato sauce
½ green pepper, diced
1½ large onions, sliced

Preheat oven to 350°. When livers are defrosted pat them partially dry. In a mixing bowl add the bran, oregano, garlic, salt and pepper. Combine them together very well. Coat the dampish livers in this mixture, coating as well as possible. In a no-stick baking dish mix the tomato sauce, green pepper, onion slices, and the rest of the dry ingredients that didn't stick to the livers. Add the coated livers to this mixture and mix well again. Bake for about 25 to 30 minutes, until livers are well cooked.

CHICKEN IN CREAM SAUCE

Fiber per serving	0.9	2 whole chicken breasts,
C/F	10.0	skinned and boned
Rating	**M, R**	½ teaspoon salt
		dash of pepper
		4 ounces tomato sauce
		1 heaping tablespoon bran
		1 clove garlic, minced
		4 ounces canned sliced
		mushrooms, drained
		½ cup cottage cheese
		¼ cup water

Put skinned chicken breasts in a hot, no-stick fry pan. Season with salt and pepper. Brown the chicken on both sides for about 10 minutes. In a small bowl combine tomato sauce, bran, garlic, and mushrooms. Pour this mixture over the chicken. Cover the pan and simmer for 20 minutes until chicken is tender. After 20 minutes uncover pan and spoon off any extra fat. Set chicken aside. Place the cottage cheese and water in a blender and mix until the cheese combination is of sour-cream consistency. Add this to the chicken. Return to stove and cook until everything is hot, about 10 minutes.

CHICKEN SENSIBLE

Fiber per serving	4.4	¾ pound mushrooms, sliced
C/F	6.4	1½ large onions, chopped
Rating	**M, R**	2 stalks celery, sliced

1   *small chicken bouillon cube*
5   *heaping tablespoons bran*
¼   *cup farmer cheese*
1   *can (5 ounce) boned*
    chicken, 2 chicken breasts,
    or 4 chicken drumsticks
    salt and pepper to taste

Put mushrooms, onions, and celery in a large covered skillet. Add half an inch of water and cook over medium heat for 10 minutes. Add the bouillon cube, bran, and cheese. Add the chicken, breaking it up into small pieces. Continue to cook on low heat for 15 minutes. Add salt and pepper if desired. Chicken breasts can be substituted if they are first stewed for about 20 minutes in a little salted water, then transferred whole to the mixture for the final 15 minutes of cooking. Use 2 breasts, one per serving, or use 4 drumsticks, 2 per serving. The R rating is maintained only if the skin is removed.

CHICKEN CRISP

Fiber per serving   **1.5**
C/F   **23.0**
Rating   **M, R**

½ *cup Grape-Nuts cereal*
2 *heaping tablespoons bran*
1 *teaspoon garlic salt*
⅛ *teaspoon pepper*
6 *tablespoons Second Nature*
  (R) = 2 eggs (M)
2 *chicken breasts, skinned and*
  boned
1 *tablespoon salad oil*

Combine cereal, bran, salt and pepper in a shallow bowl. Pour Second Nature into another bowl. Dip chicken into Second Nature, coating it well. Then dip the chicken into the cereal mixture, coating well on both sides. Place chicken in an ungreased

baking pan and sprinkle with oil. Any remaining coating mixture can be poured over chicken. Bake at 400° for 35 to 40
minutes. You can use pork chops or veal cutlets instead of
chicken and proceed the same way.

TURKEY PATTIES

Fiber per serving	**1.1**	2 heaping tablespoons bran
C/F	**9.4**	1 tablespoon whole wheat flour
Rating	**M**	½ tablespoon garlic salt
		½ tablespoon sesame seeds
		2 cans (5 ounces each) boned turkey in broth
		2 tablespoons oil

Combine all ingredients but the oil, mixing well. Form into 4
patties. Heat oil in frying pan until very hot. Fry the patties until
browned, turn and brown other side.

TUNA BAKE

Fiber per serving	**1.0**	½ cup skim milk
C/F	**13.0**	2 slices whole wheat bread, made into crumbs
Rating	**M, R**	1 can tuna (4 ounce), packed in water
		2 hard-boiled eggs, mashed salt to taste
		½ teaspoon prepared mustard
		½ teaspoon Worcestershire sauce
		dash of imitation butter flavoring
		2 teaspoons fine bran

In a bowl combine milk, bread crumbs, tuna, and mashed eggs. Add to this the salt, mustard, Worcestershire, butter flavoring, and bran. Mix all ingredients together very well. Pour mixture into a small baking dish and bake for 15 minutes at 450°.

TUNA CROQUETTES

Fiber per serving	**1.1**	*1 can (7 ounce) tuna in water,*
C/F	**4.4**	*drained*
Rating	**M, R**	*3 tablespoons Second Nature*
		(R) = 1 egg (M)
		1 heaping teaspoon garlic salt
		2 heaping tablespoons fine bran

In a bowl flake tuna into small pieces, then add all the other ingredients. Mix well. Shape tuna mixture into four patties. Place in a heated no-stick pan. Fry one side until brown. Turn and brown on other side.

MARINATED SHRIMP

Fiber per serving	**0.3**	*½ pound shrimp, raw and*
C/F	**4.7**	*washed*
Rating	**M, R**	*dietetic sweetener = 1½ tea-*
		spoons sugar
		¼ teaspoon salt
		pinch of pepper
		1 clove garlic, minced
		¼ teaspoon ginger, finely
		chopped
		1 tablespoon soy sauce
		1 teaspoon fine bran
		4 large lettuce leaves
		2 lemon wedges

Cut shrimp into ½-inch slices. Combine all other ingredients in a mixing bowl and add to shrimp. Mix together. Let stand for 30 minutes. Place 2 lettuce leaves on each plate and spoon shrimp combination onto leaves. Garnish with lemon wedge.

SHRIMP SCAMPI

Fiber per serving	1.0	2 slices whole wheat bread
C/F	14.0	1 heaping tablespoon bran
Rating	M	½ pound shrimp, raw and washed
		2 teaspoons oil
		1 clove garlic, mashed
		½ teaspoon oregano

In a blender place bread and bran. Blend until they become crumbs. Preheat oven to 350°. Line the bottom of a casserole with the raw shrimp. In a mixing bowl combine bread crumbs, oil, garlic, and oregano. Add a few drops of water to moisten. Mix this combination until well blended. Then pour over shrimp, covering them as much as possible. Place casserole in oven for about 20 minutes.

SOMETHING FISHY

Fiber per serving	4.4	¾ pound mushrooms, sliced
C/F	6.6	1½ large onions, chopped
Rating	M, R	¼ cup farmer cheese
		1 small chicken bouillon cube
		½ teaspoon imitation butter flavoring
		3 heaping tablespoons fine bran
		juice of ½ lemon
		salt and white pepper to taste

6 ounces fish, any kind, boneless
1 can (10½ ounce) asparagus,
drained, cut into 1-inch
pieces

Place the mushrooms and onions in a large covered skillet.
Add half an inch of water and cook over medium heat for 10
minutes. Add all the other ingredients except the fish and asparagus. Mix well. Push the mixture to one side of the skillet
and place the fish on the other side. Poach on low heat, covered, for 15 minutes. During the last 7 to 8 minutes add the asparagus. After the 15 minutes are up, mix well and simmer for 3
minutes. Other vegetables, such as broccoli, eggplant, or zucchini may be substituted for asparagus.

FISH AND MUSHROOMS

Fiber per serving	**1.6**	2 fillets of sole
C/F	**13.0**	1 teaspoon imitation butter fla-
Rating	**M, R**	voring

1 can (8 ounce) tomato sauce
¼ cup onion flakes
1 can (4 ounce) sliced
mushrooms, drained
1 tablespoon parsley flakes
½ teaspoon lemon juice
salt and pepper, to taste
1 heaping tablespoon bran

Preheat oven to 325°. Place raw fish slices in baking dish. Pour
imitation butter flavoring and tomato sauce over fish. Sprinkle
onion, mushrooms, parsley, lemon juice, salt, pepper, and
bran. Bake for approximately 20 to 25 minutes, or until fish is
flaky.

FRIED FISH

Fiber per serving	**1.3**	
C/F	**12.0**	
Rating	**M**	

2 heaping tablespoons bran
2 tablespoons whole wheat
   flour
1 tablespoon garlic salt
1 tablespoon sesame seeds
1 teaspoon oregano
2 fillets of flounder
2 tablespoons oil

Combine bran, flour, garlic salt, sesame seeds, and oregano in a bowl. Mix well. Dampen fish with water and dip in flour mixture, coating very well. Add oil to a frying pan and heat. Add pieces of fish and fry until browned. Turn and brown on other side.

FISH BOUILLABAISSE

Fiber per serving	**2.2**	
C/F	**5.6**	
Rating	**M, R**	

1 beef bouillon cube
½ cup water
½ teaspoon garlic, minced
½ tablespoon onion flakes
1 tablespoon green pepper,
   chopped
5 heaping tablespoons bran
2 teaspoons tomato paste
   salt and pepper, to taste
20 tiny shrimp, raw
3 ounces flounder, raw, cut into
   tiny pieces
3 ounces scallops, raw

Place bouillon cube and water in a saucepan and heat. To the pan add the garlic, onion flakes, green pepper, and bran. Stir well and bring to a boil. Boil for 10 minutes or until vegetables are tender. Add the tomato paste, salt and pepper, and cook on a lower heat for 10 minutes. Add all the seafood. Bring to a boil again. Lower heat and simmer for 15 minutes.

FISH BAKE

Fiber per serving	**2.2**	¼ pound flounder or sole, cooked
C/F	**8.6**	2 cups green beans, cooked
Rating	**M, R**	1 cup skim milk

¼ pound flounder or sole, cooked
2 cups green beans, cooked
1 cup skim milk
1 heaping tablespoon fine bran
2 slices whole wheat bread, cut in pieces
2 eggs, separated
1 teaspoon chili powder
salt to taste

Preheat oven to 350°. In a blender combine fish, green beans, milk, bran, bread, egg yolks, chili powder, and salt. Blend until perfectly smooth. Set aside. Beat the egg whites very stiff. Fold in half the fish mixture to the egg whites, and then the other half. Then pour the entire mixture into a casserole dish. Bake for 30 minutes or until browned and puffy.

ITALIAN MEAT BALLS AND SAUCE

Sauce for Meat Balls

Fiber per serving	**1.0**	½ medium onion, chopped
C/F	**13.0**	½ cup water
Rating	**M, R**	½ clove garlic, chopped

½ medium onion, chopped
½ cup water
½ clove garlic, chopped
3 ounces tomato paste
1 heaping teaspoon fine bran
1½ cup water
salt and pepper to taste

Cook onions in water in covered skillet until tender and excess water is gone. Add the garlic and cook 1 minute more. Add tomato paste, bran, and water. Stir until well blended. Add salt and pepper to taste and simmer uncovered for 1 hour. While simmering, prepare meatballs.

Italian Meat Balls

Fiber per serving	**0.9**	
C/F	**5.0**	
Rating	**M, R**	

3 tablespoons Second Nature (R) = 1 egg (M), slightly beaten
½ pound ground beef
2 tablespoons bran
2 tablespoons water or beef stock
1 tablespoon onions, chopped
1 tablespoon parmesan cheese, grated
salt and pepper to taste
¼ teaspoon garlic powder
¼ teaspoon oregano

In a mixing bowl, combine all ingredients and mix completely. Shape into small balls. Place balls in boiling tomato sauce and cook slowly for about 25 minutes, until meat balls are cooked.

SPAGHETTI SAUCE

Fiber per serving	**4.2**	
C/F	**13.0**	
Rating	**M, R**	

3 medium onions, chopped fine
¼ pound ground beef
14 ounces whole peeled tomatoes, Italian style (from a 28 ounce can)
1 can (6 ounce) tomato paste

½ *garlic clove, minced*
½ *teaspoon oregano*
1 *teaspoon black pepper*
2 *heaping tablespoons bran*

Put onions, meat, and whole peeled tomatoes in a large saucepan. Simmer until the onions are soft and the meat is browned. Add tomato paste, minced garlic, oregano, pepper and bran. Mix well. Cover tightly and simmer on low heat for 1 hour, stirring occasionally. Serve hot over whole wheat spaghetti.

ITALIAN MEAT DELIGHT

Fiber per serving	**5.4**	¾ *pound mushrooms, sliced*
C/F	**6.8**	1½ *large onions, chopped*
Rating	**M, R**	1 *large green pepper, chopped*
		¼ *cup farmer cheese*
		3 *ounces tomato paste*
		1 *teaspoon Marmite*
		1 *teaspoon Italian seasoning garlic salt to taste pepper to taste red pepper (optional)*
		5 *heaping tablespoons bran*
		¼ *pound lean ground beef*

Place mushrooms, onions, and green pepper in a large covered skillet. Add half an inch of water and cook over medium heat for 10 minutes. Add the farmer cheese, tomato paste, Marmite, Italian seasoning, garlic salt, pepper, and red pepper if desired. Cook on medium heat for about 5 minutes more and then add the bran. Add the meat, breaking it up with constant mashing and stirring. Simmer on low heat for about 15 minutes and serve.

VEAL SCALLOPINE WITH MUSHROOMS

Fiber per serving	1.7
C/F	4.7
Rating	M, R

½ pound boneless veal cutlets, sliced very thin
1 teaspoon salt
1 teaspoon pepper
2 heaping tablespoons bran
½ clove garlic, minced
1 bay leaf
1 teaspoon lemon juice
1 tablespoon margarine
½ pound mushrooms, sliced

Ask your butcher to slice the veal very thin. On a plate, season the veal with salt and pepper. Then coat veal with bran. Cover both sides as heavily as possible. Heat a no-stick fry pan, sprayed with vegetable coating. When pan is hot add minced garlic and brown slightly. Add bay leaf to browning garlic. Immediately add the veal slices and brown the meat with the garlic and bay leaf over a medium-high heat until the meat is browned well—about 1 minute on each side. When meat is browned remove it and the bay leaf. Place meat on a serving platter. Throw the bay leaf away. Add the lemon juice to the pan and scrape pan to gather up the bits of meat. Pour scrapings, lemon juice, and garlic over meat. In the same skillet melt the 1 tablespoon margarine, then add the mushrooms and sauté them for about 4 minutes on medium heat. Pour this mixture over veal. Serve immediately.

VEAL AND PEPPERS

Fiber per serving	3.0
C/F	5.7
Rating	M

1 large green pepper, cut in strips
½ medium red pepper, cut in strips
2 tablespoons oil
½ pound boneless veal cutlets, sliced thin and in strips

1 can (4 ounce) sliced
mushrooms, drained
1 can (8 ounce) tomato sauce
1 heaping tablespoon fine bran
salt and pepper to taste

Preheat oven to 325°. In a frying pan sauté green and red peppers in oil for about 10 minutes. When they are tender, remove
them from the oil. Drain on a paper towel. Use the same pan to
cook the veal. Brown it on both sides, about 5 minutes each
side. Next add the mushrooms and cook about 5 to 7 minutes,
until mushrooms are soft. Add tomato sauce, bran, salt and
pepper, and mix well. Pour all the ingredients from the pan,
plus the peppers, into a 1-quart casserole and mix together.
Cover it with a piece of aluminum foil and bake for 1 hour at
325°.

CELERY PARMIGIANA

Fiber per serving	**2.4**	
C/F	**8.3**	
Rating	**M, R**	

1 cup water
1 chicken bouillon cube
6 stalks celery, cut in pieces 3
inches long by ¼ inch wide
½ cup tomato paste
3 ounces mozzarella cheese,
thinly sliced
2 tablespoons fine bran
onion salt to taste
2 tablespoons parmesan
cheese

Boil the water in a small saucepan. Add the bouillon cube and
dissolve it. Add the celery, cover, and cook until just tender,
about 15 minutes. After cooking, transfer half the celery from
the bouillon into a shallow casserole. Cover with a third of the
tomato paste and half the mozzarella cheese, and sprinkle on
bran and onion salt. Repeat layers, ending with tomato paste.
Top with parmesan cheese. Bake at 400° for 15 minutes, until
hot and bubbly.

EGGPLANT PARMESAN

Fiber per serving	**2.8**
C/F	**15.0**
Rating	**M**

½ *medium eggplant, peeled and sliced thin*
1 *teaspoon salt*
½ *cup whole wheat flour*
1 *heaping tablespoon bran*
½ *teaspoon dried oregano, chopped*
  salt and pepper to taste
1 *clove garlic, chopped*
1 *tablespoon cooking oil*
4 *tablespoons water*
3 *ounces tomato paste*
3 *ounces mozzarella cheese, cut in slices*
3 *tablespoons parmesan cheese, grated*

Preheat oven to 350°. Place sliced eggplant on a platter with the slices separated. Sprinkle slices with salt and set aside. In a medium size bowl place whole wheat flour, bran, oregano, salt, pepper, and garlic. Mix well together. Add the oil to a frying pan and heat until very hot. While oil is heating up, dip the pieces of eggplant into flour mixture. Coat the eggplant pieces very well on both sides. When the pieces are coated, fry them in hot oil and brown one side for about 3 minutes. Then turn and brown other side. Remove eggplant and drain on a paper towel. Place the pieces of the eggplant on the bottom of a 1-quart casserole or baking dish. In a separate bowl combine water and tomato paste. Mix together and spread evenly over the eggplant slices. Next place cut slices of mozzarella cheese evenly over sauce and sprinkle on the parmesan cheese. Bake uncovered for 25 to 30 minutes.

BEEF MARINADE

Fiber per serving	1.1
C/F	7.4
Rating	**M, R**

1 pound flank steak, partially
    frozen
¼ cup soy sauce
1 tablespoon onion, minced
½ clove garlic, minced
1 heaping tablespoon fine bran
¼ cup scallions, chopped
2 tablespoons sesame seeds

Cut partially frozen steak into bite size pieces. In a mixing bowl add meat, soy sauce, onion, garlic, and bran. Mix together and cover. Place in refrigerator for two hours. *Two hours later:* Heat a large no-stick skillet. Add just the meat from marinade to skillet and pan-fry the pieces until they are seared. When cooked to desired doneness, place meat on serving platter. Put marinade into pan. Add scallions and heat until bubbly. Toast sesame seeds on a piece of foil for two minutes. Pour marinade mixture over meat and sprinkle with sesame seeds.

MEAT LOAF

Fiber per serving	3.4
C/F	11.2
Rating	**M, R**

1 cup ground beef
½ cup fresh mushrooms, sliced,
    or 1 can (4 ounce) sliced
    mushrooms, drained
2 tablespoons onion flakes
3 tablespoons Second Nature
    (R) = 1 egg (M)
3 tablespoons bran
½ teaspoon garlic salt
¼ cup tomato sauce
⅛ teaspoon Marmite

Combine all ingredients. Mix well and shape into loaf. Put in loaf pan. Bake at 350° for 1 hour for well-done meat loaf, less time for rarer loaf.

GROUND BEEF GOULASH

Fiber per serving	1.9
C/F	8.3
Rating	M

½ pound egg whole wheat soy noodles (obtainable in health food stores)
½ pound ground beef
2 heaping tablespoons fine bran
1 egg, beaten
½ teaspoon salt
⅛ teaspoon pepper
½ tablespoon onion flakes
⅛ teaspoon thyme
⅛ teaspoon Marmite
5½ ounces tomato soup (canned, condensed)
3 ounces V-8 vegetable juice
3 tablespoons cheddar cheese, shredded

Cook noodles according to package directions. In a mixing bowl combine ground beef, bran, egg, salt, pepper, onion flakes, thyme, and Marmite. Mix very well. Shape mixture into 12 meatballs. Heat a no-stick fry pan and brown meatballs on all sides. Then place meatballs in a 1-quart casserole. Add the soup, juice, and noodles. Mix all together. Place in oven and bake for 30 minutes at 400°. Remove and add cheese, and cook for another 5 to 8 minutes, until cheese melts.

MOUSSAKA

Fiber per serving	**3.0**
C/F	**6.7**
Rating	**M, R**

½ medium eggplant, cut in
   ½-inch slices
   salt
½ pound ground beef
1 heaping tablespoon fine bran
⅛ teaspoon Marmite
1 cup tomato juice, reduced to
   half by boiling
1 tablespoon dried onion flakes
½ teaspoon lemon rind, grated
1 clove garlic, crushed
½ teaspoon salt
¼ teaspoon pepper
   White Sauce With Cauliflower
   (next recipe)

Sprinkle eggplant pieces with salt. Let stand for about 30 minutes to remove excess water. In a no-stick frying pan brown meat. Add bran, Marmite, thickened tomato juice, onion flakes, lemon rind, garlic, salt and pepper. Mix all very well. Pour meat mixture into a shallow baking dish or casserole. Dry off eggplant with a paper towel and place eggplant pieces over meat mixture. Spoon White Sauce With Cauliflower on top. Bake covered for 30 minutes at 375°.

White Sauce with Cauliflower

1 cup skim milk
2 cups frozen cauliflower, defrosted
½ teaspoon salt
½ teaspoon imitation butter flavoring
1 teaspoon fine bran

In a small saucepan simmer milk. Add the defrosted cauliflower florets and cook until they are very soft. Place this combination in a blender. Add salt, butter flavoring, and bran. Purée until sauce is creamy. If sauce is too thick add a few drops of water. Delicious on Moussaka.

BEEF AND ZUCCHINI

Fiber per serving	3.3	
C/F	6.1	
Rating	M, R	

1 tablespoon oil
½ medium onion, diced
½ medium green pepper, diced
½ pound ground beef
2 medium zucchini, sliced in
   1-inch pieces
   salt and pepper to taste
8 ounces Italian-style whole
   peeled tomatoes
1 heaping tablespoon fine bran

Put oil in a large frying pan and heat until hot. Add onions and peppers and sauté them until they are crisp. Add the ground beef and cook the meat until it is browned. When the meat is browned, carefully add the pieces of zucchini. Blend the zucchini with the ingredients in the pan. Stir in the salt and pepper. Pour in the whole peeled tomatoes and bran. Stir all together. Pour the entire mixture into a 1-quart casserole. Bake uncovered for 30 minutes at 350°.

TASTY BURGERS

Fiber per serving	0.6
C/F	5.4
Rating	M, R

½ pound ground beef or veal
1 tablespoon Second Nature
  (R) = ⅓ egg, beaten (M)
1 tablespoon water
¼ teaspoon garlic, minced
½ teaspoon onion flakes
⅛ teaspoon pepper
½ teaspoon poppy seeds
  pinch of crushed red pepper
¼ teaspoon oregano
2 heaping teaspoons fine bran

Combine all ingredients and mix well. Shape meat into 4 patties and fry in no-stick skillet sprayed with vegetable coating.

MEATBALLS WITH PEANUTS

Fiber per serving	1.5
C/F	9.3
Rating	M, R

3 tablespoons Second Nature
  (R) =1 egg (M)
¼ cup skim milk
3 heaping tablespoons bran
½ teaspoon salt
  pinch of pepper
½ pound chopped meat
¼ cup peanuts, chopped
¾ cup water
½ envelope (½ ounce package)
  onion gravy mix
1 teaspoon curry or chili
  powder

Combine Second Nature, milk, bran, salt, and pepper. Add meat and two tablespoons of peanuts. Mix together. Shape into 6 meatballs. In a no-stick pan brown meatballs on all sides.

Then add the water, gravy mix, and curry or chili powder. Bring to a boil, then reduce heat and simmer for about 10 minutes. Add the rest of the peanuts. Serve with noodles or mashed potatoes.

UNSTUFFED CABBAGE

Cabbage Rolls

Fiber per serving	4.7
C/F	6.0
Rating	M, R

½ pound ground beef
2 heaping tablespoons fine bran
½ medium onion, grated
3 tablespoons Second Nature (R) = 1 egg (M)
salt and pepper to taste
1 medium cabbage, separated into leaves
1 can (8 ounce) sauerkraut, drained

Combine in a bowl the meat, bran, onion, Second Nature, salt and pepper. Mix all ingredients very well and shape into 1-inch round meatballs. Place a third of the cabbage, a third of the meat balls, and a third of the sauerkraut in layers in a 1-quart casserole. Repeat this process three times. Then pour Sauce (below) over this mixture.

Sauce

4 ounces tomato sauce
1 tablespoon vinegar
½ cup water
½ cup raisins (optional)

Mix all together. Pour over cabbage and meat and sauerkraut combination. Bake 1½ hours at 350°.

SWEET AND SOUR
STUFFED CABBAGE

Fiber per serving	3.7	
C/F	7.0	
Rating	**M, R**	

½   large head of cabbage
½   teaspoon salt
2   cups water, boiling
¼   medium onion, chopped
½   cup water
3   tablespoons fine bran
½   teaspoon salt
¼   teaspoon cinnamon
⅛   teaspoon pepper
3   tablespoons Second Nature
      (R) = 1 egg (M)
1½ tablespoons water
½   pound ground beef

Separate cabbage leaves and place them in a large saucepan.
Sprinkle leaves with ½ teaspoon salt. Pour 2 cups boiling water
over leaves. Boil for 3 minutes. Then drain and set leaves aside.
In another saucepan saute the onions in ½ cup water. When
onions are soft add bran, salt, cinnamon, and pepper. Mix very
well. In another bowl add Second Nature, 1½ tablespoons
water and ground beef and mix well. Add this combination to
the onion mixture. Mix all together. Divide mixture into 6 portions and set aside.

Stuffed Cabbage Sauce

1   medium onion, diced
4   tablespoons tomato paste
      artificial sweetener = 2 table-
      spoons sugar
⅛   teaspoon ginger
⅛   teaspoon allspice
¼   teaspoon lemon juice
¼   cup beef broth (canned)

In a bowl combine all ingredients. Mix together and set aside.

To Stuff Cabbage: Spread out individual cabbage leaves. Place a portion of meat mixture in each flattened leaf. Roll leaf around filling and place open end down in casserole. Secure with a toothpick. Pour sauce over cabbages stuffed with meat, soaking each one very well. Bake 1 hour at 350°.

BEEF STEW CHINESE STYLE

Fiber per serving	**1.7**	
C/F	**10.0**	
Rating	**M, R**	

1 tablespoon whole wheat flour
½ teaspoon salt
1 pound lean chuck, cut into 1-inch cubes
¼ cup water
½ medium onion, thin sliced
1 stalk celery, cut in 1-inch pieces
¼ cup scallions, cut in pieces
½ can (8½ ounce) water chestnuts, cut in small pieces
½ cup canned sliced mushrooms, drained
1 heaping tablespoon fine bran

Combine flour and salt in a shallow bowl. Dip meat into flour mixture, coating well. In a no-stick fry pan, brown all sides of the meat. Then cover pan and cook very slowly. After 5 minutes add ¼ cup water to prevent sticking. Cook until meat is tender, about 15 minutes. When meat is tender, add all the vegetables and the bran. Cook uncovered until the vegetables are tender but crisp, about 10 minutes.

CHINESE-STYLE GREEN PEPPER AND CABBAGE

Fiber per serving	**3.1**
C/F	**5.0**
Rating	**M, R**

½ cup water
½ medium cabbage, shredded
1 medium green pepper, chopped
½ medium onion, chopped
¼ teaspoon salt
¼ teaspoon pepper
3 ounces chicken broth
1 heaping teaspoon fine bran
dietetic sweetener = 6 table-spoons sugar
½ tablespoon vinegar

Place water in a medium size saucepan. Add cabbage, green pepper, and onions. Cover pot and simmer until ingredients are tender. Stir with a fork. Season with salt and pepper. Add chicken broth and mix well. Add bran, sweetener, and vinegar. Mix very well. Cover and cook for 5 minutes. Stir and serve hot.

CHINESE EGGS

Fiber per serving	**0.6**
C/F	**5.9**
Rating	**M, R**

1 stalk celery, diced
2 tablespoons onion flakes
2 tablespoons pepper flakes
1 cup water
2 tablespoons canned bean sprouts, drained
12 tablespoons Second Nature (R) = 4 eggs (M)
1 heaping teaspoon fine bran
salt and pepper to taste
soy sauce to taste

Put celery, onion, and pepper flakes into a saucepan. Add 1 cup of water. Cook covered until celery is soft, about 15 minutes. Then add the bean sprouts. Mix well. In a small bowl add Second Nature to the bran. Add salt and pepper to taste and mix well. Drain the vegetables and add them to the eggs. Mix well. Heat a no-stick fry pan and pour mixture in. Scramble mixture until eggs are cooked. Remove and put on platter. Serve with soy sauce.

TEMPURA BATTER
(Can be used for frying shrimp, onion rings, cauliflower, broccoli, and carrots)

Fiber per serving	**1.5**	¼ cup whole wheat flour
C/F	**11.0**	2 heaping tablespoons fine
Rating	**M**	bran
		¼ cup ice water
		½ egg, beaten
		1 tablespoon oil
		dietetic sweetener = 1 teaspoon sugar
		¼ teaspoon salt

In a mixing bowl mix all ingredients until well moistened. Keep the batter cool by putting one ice cube into it. Dip the food to be coated into batter. Cover well with mixture. Fry in deep fat (360°) until the surfaces of food are browned. Drain well. Serve at once.

CHEESE AND MUSHROOM QUICHE

Fiber per serving	**2.0**	1 pie crust (see p. 222)
C/F	**15.0**	1 tablespoon whole wheat flour
Rating	**M**	¾ cup cheddar cheese, shredded

1 egg
½ cup skim milk
¼ teaspoon salt
¼ teaspoon pepper
1 heaping tablespoon fine bran
1 cup fresh mushrooms, sliced

Make pie crust. Set aside. Place the flour and cheddar cheese in a bowl. Mix together. Add egg, milk, and all the remaining ingredients except the mushrooms. Mix very well. Fold in the sliced mushrooms. Pour mixture into pie crust. Bake in a 350° oven for 45 minutes.

BRAN BALLS AND SAUCE

Fiber per serving	3.0	
C/F	7.5	
Rating	M, R	

4 heaping tablespoons bran
6 tablespoons Second Nature
  (R) = 2 eggs (M)
2 tablespoons onion soup mix
⅛ teaspoon Marmite
1 can (8 ounce) tomato sauce
½ cup water
½ green pepper, sliced
1 teaspoon celery salt
  salt and pepper to taste

In a mixing bowl combine bran, Second Nature, onion soup mix, and Marmite. Mix well and form into 1-inch round balls. Set aside. In a saucepan add tomato sauce, water, green pepper, celery salt, salt and pepper. Stir well. Allow to boil. When sauce boils, lower heat to simmer. Add bran balls to sauce. Cover and cook for about 20 minutes.

VEGETABLES

ACORN SQUASH

Fiber per serving	1.8	1 medium acorn squash
C/F	5.7	salt
Rating	**M**	¼ cup margarine
		dietetic brown sugar = 12 teaspoons brown sugar
		1 tablespoon cinnamon
		1 heaping teaspoon fine bran

Cut squash lengthwise and remove seeds and rind. Place upside down on a piece of aluminum foil or cookie sheet. Bake for 30 minutes in a 375° oven. Turn squash over. Fill each cavity with sprinkle of salt, half of the margarine, half each of the dietetic brown sugar, cinnamon, and bran. Return both halves to oven and bake 15 minutes more, or until squash is tender.

TASTY BEANS

Fiber per serving	2.6	½ tablespoon oil
C/F	6.9	½ medium onion, chopped
Rating	**M, R**	½ clove garlic, minced
		1 medium tomato, diced
		½ teaspoon green pepper, minced
		½ teaspoon parsley flakes
		salt and pepper to taste
		1 heaping tablespoon fine bran
		1 package (10 ounce) frozen green beans, cooked and drained

Heat oil in a frying pan until hot. Add onion and garlic and sauté until tender, about 3 to 5 minutes. In a serving bowl mix tomatoes, green pepper, parsley, salt, pepper, and bran. Add sautéed garlic and onion to this mixture, including its oil. Then add cooked hot green beans. Mix together very well. Serve hot.

SAUTÉED BROCCOLI

Fiber per serving	2.6	½ medium fresh broccoli
C/F	3.2	1 tablespoon oil
Rating	**M, R**	⅛ teaspoon dry mustard
		1 heaping tablespoon bran
		1 cup water
		½ tablespoon salt
		1 tablespoon powdered bouillon

Wash broccoli and cut in small pieces. In a fry pan heat the oil and add the mustard. Stir well. Add pieces of broccoli and the bran. Sauté for about 2 minutes, mixing well. Add water, salt, and powdered bouillon. Stir gently. Cover and cook for about 10 minutes.

CARROTS LYONNAISE

Fiber per serving	2.8	3 medium carrots, raw
C/F	10.0	⅓ cup water, boiling
Rating	**M**	1 bouillon cube (beef or chicken)
		3 tablespoons margarine or butter
		1 medium onion, sliced in rings and separated
		1 tablespoon whole wheat flour
		1 tablespoon fine bran
		salt and pepper to taste

Wash and pare carrots. Slice carrots into 1-inch pieces. In a small saucepan add the boiling water and bouillon cube. Dissolve cube in water. Add the carrots and cook for about 20 minutes, until they are soft. In another saucepan melt the margarine over low heat. Add the onion rings. Cover pan and cook for about 10 minutes, until onions are soft. Next, add flour, bran, salt and pepper. Mix well and bring to a boil. Lower heat and cook uncovered for about 5 minutes. Stir well before serving.

CAULIFLOWER AU GRATIN

Cauliflower

Fiber per serving	**2.1**	½ *medium cauliflower*
C/F	**4.5**	½ *cup water*
Rating	**M, R**	¼ *teaspoon salt*

Separate cauliflower into pieces. In a saucepan boil the water and add the salt. Add the cauliflower and cover pot. Cook for about 10 minutes. Drain and save liquid for Sauce. Place cauliflower in casserole.

Sauce

2   *tablespoons water*
½   *medium onion, minced*
1½ *tablespoons cottage cheese cooking liquid (from cauliflower) plus enough skim milk to make ¾ cup*
1   *tablespoon diet margarine salt and pepper, to taste*

In a small saucepan place 2 tablespoons water and onions.

Cook until onions are transparent. Add cottage cheese and stir. Cook until mixture bubbles. Gradually add cooking liquid (with milk) and margarine. Boil until mixture thickens. Add salt and pepper. Pour over cauliflower.

Topping

4 *heaping teaspoons bran*
1 *tablespoon parmesan cheese, grated*
1 *tablespoon diet margarine*

Combine bran and cheese in small bowl. Sprinkle over cauliflower casserole and dot with margarine. Bake for 15 minutes at 375°.

CORN CASSEROLE

Fiber per serving	**2.6**	1 *cup skim milk*
C/F	**9.4**	1 *cup canned corn kernels,*
Rating	**M, R**	*drained*

1 *heaping teaspoon fine bran*
½ *medium onion, chopped*
1 *green pepper, chopped*
3 *tablespoons Second Nature (R) = 1 egg (M)*
1 *teaspoon butter-flavored salt dash of pepper*

Preheat oven to 325°. In a medium saucepan, scald the milk. Drain the corn and add along with the other ingredients to the scalded milk. Stir together. Place mixture in 1-quart casserole and bake for 30 minutes.

EGGPLANT DELICACIES

Fiber per serving	1.0	4 *slices peeled eggplant,*
C/F	4.6	*¼-inch thick*
Rating	**M, R**	4 *slices tomato, thin sliced*
		4 *slices skim milk mozzarella cheese, ⅛-inch thick*
		4 *small slices green pepper*
		dash of garlic salt
		2 *heaping teaspoons fine bran*

On each slice of eggplant place a piece of tomato, a slice of mozzarella cheese, a slice of green pepper, dash of garlic salt, and ½ teaspoon bran. Place eggplant slices on a piece of aluminum foil and bake for about 10 minutes until tomato softens and cheese melts and becomes bubbly.

KASHA
(Buckwheat Groats and Bran)

Fiber per serving	0.6	¼ *cup buckwheat groats*
(3 heaping		¾ *cup bran*
tablespoons)		1 *egg, beaten*
C/F	10.0	2½ *cups water, boiling*
Rating	**M, R**	

Mix buckwheat groats and bran. Add egg and mix thoroughly. Place in dry skillet and heat, constantly breaking up lumps, until grains are dry and separate. Add boiling water to skillet. Cover and simmer for 30 minutes. A serving of three heaping tablespoons provides the amount of fiber listed above. Serving size is variable.

NOODLE PUDDING

Fiber per serving	**3.3**	2 cups water, boiling
C/F	**23.0**	6 ounces whole wheat egg
Rating	**M**	noodles

2 eggs
½ cup skim milk
½ cup orange juice
½ teaspoon salt
¼ teaspoon pepper
⅓ cup parmesan cheese, grated
2 tablespoons fine bran

Cook noodles in boiling water for 10 to 12 minutes. Drain noodles in a strainer or colander. Rinse in cool water. Pour noodles into a no-stick 1-quart casserole. Beat eggs well and combine them with milk and orange juice. Add the salt, pepper, parmesan cheese, and bran. Mix together and pour mixture over noodles and combine well. Bake in 350° oven for 1 hour.

QUICK MASHED POTATOES

Fiber per serving	**0.9**	1 heaping tablespoon fine bran
C/F	**20.0**	¾ cup water
Rating	**M**	⅔ cup mashed potato mix

1 tablespoon butter or margarine
¼ teaspoon salt
¼ cup milk
minced onion flakes (optional)

Follow instructions on the mashed potato mix package for making 2 servings, except use 50 percent more water than called for. For example, if the instructions call for a ½ cup of water, use ¾ cup. Mix the bran with the water then follow the rest of the directions. Add minced onion flakes for a variation.

REAL MASHED POTATOES

Fiber per serving	1.1	*1 heaping tablespoon fine bran*
C/F	18.0	*½ cup water*
Rating	**M**	*2 medium potatoes, peeled, quartered, and boiled*
		3 tablespoons butter
		3 tablespoons milk
		salt and pepper to taste

Gently boil bran in ½ cup water until water is almost gone. Be very careful not to burn the bran. Drain and set aside. Mash potatoes with butter and milk. Add the bran and mix well. Salt and pepper to taste.

POTATO STUFFERS

Fiber per serving	1.9	*2 large baking potatoes*
C/F	25.0	*2 tablespoons milk, hot*
Rating	**M**	*1 heaping tablespoon fine bran*
		1 teaspoon onion salt
		¼ teaspoon pepper
		dash of paprika

Bake potatoes in a hot oven for 1 hour, until they are soft. Cut potatoes in half lengthwise and scoop out the inside, leaving skin whole. Mash potato insides, adding the hot milk, bran, onion salt, and pepper. Divide mixture between potato shells

and fill shells. Sprinkle a little paprika on each potato. About 15
to 20 minutes before use, put potatoes in a shallow baking pan
and bake at 400°.

SPINACH SAUTÉED WITH GARLIC

Fiber per serving	**1.3**	½ pound fresh spinach, chopped
C/F	**5.4**	½ clove garlic, crushed
Rating	**M, R**	¼ teaspoon salt
		1 heaping tablespoon bran
		1 tablespoon oil

Wash, drain, and dry spinach very well. Place in a salad bowl.
Add garlic, salt, and bran. Mix and toss thoroughly. Heat oil in a
frying pan. When oil is hot, add spinach combination and sauté
for about 3 to 5 minutes. Stir mixture carefully with a fork.
Serve hot.

MUSHROOM AND SPINACH COMBO

Fiber per serving	**3.0**	1 package (16 ounce) frozen chopped spinach, defrosted
C/F	**4.2**	1 cup chicken broth, canned
Rating	**M, R**	½ tablespoon onion flakes
		2 heaping teaspoons bran
		6 large fresh mushrooms, sliced
		salt and pepper to taste

In a saucepan simmer the spinach in the chicken broth. Add
the minced onions and the bran. When spinach is soft, add

mushrooms and heat for 5 minutes. Add salt and pepper to taste.

STUFFED TOMATOES

Fiber per serving	3.0
C/F	7.5
Rating	**M, R**

1 package (10 ounce) frozen green beans, cooked and cooled
2 ounces canned sliced mushrooms, drained
2 tablespoons low-calorie Italian dressing
2 tablespoons scallions, sliced
dash of salt and pepper
1 heaping tablespoon fine bran
2 tablespoons green pepper, chopped fine
2 medium tomatoes, centers removed

In a mixing bowl combine first seven ingredients. Mix very well together. Set aside. Remove centers of tomatoes, leaving a casing about one-half to one inch thick. Place equal amounts of vegetable combination in each tomato shell, piling them high. Chill until ready to serve.

HOT VEGETABLE SALAD WITH NUTS

Fiber per serving	4.7
C/F	9.5
Rating	**M, R**

½ tablespoon margarine
⅛ teaspoon oregano
½ teaspoon salt
1 tablespoon bran
½ cup chopped walnuts

½ cup diet Italian dressing
2 cooked carrots, cut in 1-inch
  pieces
1 package (9 ounce) frozen
  green beans, cooked and
  drained
1 package (10 ounce) frozen
  cauliflower, cooked and
  drained

Melt the margarine in a saucepan. Add the oregano, salt, bran, and nuts. Stir well. Cook over medium heat for 5 to 7 minutes, until nuts start to brown. In another saucepan heat the Italian salad dressing.

On a platter arrange the cooked hot vegetables in separate clumps of carrots, green beans, and cauliflower. Pour the buttered nuts over vegetables, then pour the heated dressing over nuts and vegetables. Serve piping hot.

VEGETABLE STUFFING

Fiber per serving	2.3	
C/F	9.0	
Rating	**M, R**	

¼ pound mushrooms, chopped
  fine
1 carrot, shredded
1 celery stalk, diced
1 medium onion, diced
¼ cup skim milk
½ tablespoon parsley flakes
1 heaping tablespoon fine bran
  salt and pepper to taste

In a no-stick saucepan add all the ingredients and cook over low heat for 5 minutes. Then cover pan and simmer for 30 minutes. Stir frequently. When done it can be used as a side dish or to stuff a small chicken.

STUFFING

Fiber per serving	**1.1**	¾ cup water
C/F	**15.0**	1 chicken bouillon cube
Rating	**M, R**	1 stalk celery, diced
		½ large onion, chopped fine
		2 slices whole wheat bread, made into bread crumbs (see p. 230)
		seasonings to taste
		1 teaspoon salt
		pinch of pepper
		1 heaping teaspoon fine bran

Put water in a saucepan and bring to a boil. Add bouillon cube and dissolve. Add celery and onion and cook until they are soft and the bouillon is almost evaporated, about 15 minutes. While onion and celery are cooking, place bread crumbs in a bowl and add seasonings, salt, pepper, and bran. Mix well. Add mixture to cooked celery combination. This stuffing can be used to stuff chicken or turkey, or stuffed into tomato or green pepper shells.

BREADS

PERFECTLY HEALTHY BREAD

Fiber per serving	**0.7**	dietetic sweetener = 30 teaspoons sugar
(1 very thin slice, ³/₁₆ inch)		
C/F	**20.0**	2 packages dry yeast (each ¼ ounce)
Rating	**M, T**	4 cups water, warm but not hot

5½ cups unsifted whole wheat
flour
2 cups gluten flour
1 cup finely ground bran
2 tablespoons cooking oil
1 teaspoon salt

Dissolve sweetener and yeast in warm water in a large bowl. All lumps must be dissolved. Add 3½ cups whole wheat flour, 1 cup gluten flour, and the bran. Mix thoroughly. Cover with a towel and let rise in a warm place for about 1 hour or until doubled in volume. Add oil and salt, and 1½ cups whole wheat flour and 1 cup gluten flour. Begin to knead. If dough is sticky, add a little more whole wheat flour. Knead for 10 to 12 minutes. Let rise again as before. Work dough down in size. Divide into two pieces. Shape into loaves and place in 2 lightly greased 9"-loaf pans. Bake for about 1 hour in preheated 350° oven.

APPLE MUFFINS

Fiber per serving	**2.0**	
C/F	**15.0**	
Rating	**M, R**	

2 slices whole wheat bread,
well toasted
2 medium apples, peeled,
cored, and grated
6 tablespoons Second Nature
(R) = 2 eggs (M)
dietetic sweetener = 6 teaspoons sugar
⅓ teaspoon orange extract
⅓ teaspoon vanilla extract
¼ teaspoon cinnamon
1 heaping teaspoon fine bran

Break toasted bread into pieces and put them in a blender. Make bread crumbs (see page 230). Put crumbs in a bowl and add grated apples. Add all the remaining ingredients and stir well. Spoon into a no-stick muffin pan. Bake in a 375° oven, not preheated, for about 35 minutes.

BRAN MUFFINS

Fiber per serving	**1.2**	½ cup whole wheat flour
C/F	**21.0**	1½ teaspoons baking powder
Rating	**M**	¼ teaspoon salt
		1 tablespoon bran
		½ egg
		dietetic sweetener = 6 teaspoons sugar
		½ cup skim milk
		1 tablespoon oil

Heat oven to 425°. Combine flour, baking powder, and salt. Add the bran and mix well. Next add the egg, sweetener, milk, and oil. Mix well, so that entire mixture is moistened. Fill no-stick muffin pans ⅔ full with mixture. Bake approximately 15 minutes. For added zing, you can add ½ cup raisins or ½ cup walnuts.

DESSERTS

BAKED APPLES

Fiber per serving	**2.6**	2 large baking apples
C/F	**12.0**	¾ cup dietetic black cherry soda
Rating	**M, R**	dietetic sweetener = 3 teaspoons sugar
		1 tablespoon cinnamon
		1 heaping tablespoon fine bran

Core apples and place them in a small baking dish. Combine
the soda, sweetener, cinnamon, and bran in a bowl. Pour equal
portions over apples and let remainder of the juice spill into
baking pan so you can baste as the apples are cooking. If
apples are large or if you like them soft, bake for 1 hour at 350°.
If apples are small or medium, or if you like them firmer, bake
for 30 to 45 minutes at 350°. Baste every 15 minutes to ensure a
soft, moist apple.

APPLESAUCE PASTRIES

Fiber per serving	1.3	2 *slices whole wheat bread*
C/F	17.0	1 *teaspoon cinnamon*
Rating	**M, R**	*dietetic sweetener* = 1 *table-spoon sugar*
		1 *heaping teaspoon fine bran*
		1 *cup Applesauce* (next recipe)

Put oven on broil. Remove crusts from bread and with a rolling
pin roll bread very thin. Combine cinnamon, sweetener, and
bran, and sprinkle pieces of bread with a small amount of this
mixture. Place half the applesauce on one side (triangle) of
each piece of bread. Fold the bread in a triangle. Pinch the
edges tightly all the way around so the applesauce stays inside
bread. Sprinkle tops of bread with some more cinnamon,
sweetener, and bran mixture. Put the bread on a piece of aluminum foil and broil lightly. Turn, sprinkle other side with more
mixture, and broil again. Be sure to turn carefully.

HOMEMADE APPLESAUCE

Fiber per serving	2.3
C/F	14.0
Rating	M, R

3 apples, cut in pieces (don't
   peel or core)
½ cup cherry-flavored diet soda
½ teaspoon cinnamon
⅛ teaspoon grated lemon rind
   dietetic sweetener = 3 teaspoons sugar

Mix all ingredients except sweetener in a saucepan. Bring mixture to a boil. Lower heat and simmer until apples are soft.
Remove from the heat, then add sweetener and mix well. Put
mixture through a strainer. Taste and add more sweetener if
necessary. Chill.

BANANA FRITTERS

Fiber per serving	1.4
C/F	22.0
Rating	M, R

2 ripe bananas
6 tablespoons Second Nature
   (R) = 2 eggs (M)
2 slices whole wheat bread, cut
   in pieces
¼ teaspoon orange extract
2 tablespoons water
   artificial sweetener = 5 teaspoons sugar
   dash of cinnamon
1 teaspoon fine bran

In a bowl mash bananas very well and set aside. Combine all
the other ingredients in a blender or electric mixer or a mixing
bowl. Beat or blend until mixture is very smooth. Fold in the
banana. Mix very well. Drop mixture by the tablespoon into a

hot no-stick skillet sprayed with no-stick spray. Cook on both
sides to a golden brown.

CRÊPES

Fiber per serving	**2.0**	2 slices whole wheat bread
C/F	**15.0**	2 tablespoons water
Rating	**M, R**	6 tablespoons Second Nature

6 tablespoons Second Nature
(R) = 2 eggs (M)
¼ teaspoon rum extract
1 heaping teaspoon fine bran
dietetic sweetener = 4 teaspoons sugar
Fruit Filling (next recipe)

In a blender combine bread, water, egg substitute, rum flavoring, bran, and sweetener. Blend until mixture is very smooth. In
a hot no-stick pan, sprayed with no-stick vegetable coating,
pour in half of the batter. Cook until batter starts to bubble.
Turn and brown on other side. Repeat with other half of batter.
Keep crêpes warm and prepare filling.

Fruit Filling

2 medium apples, peeled,
pared, and diced
2 tablespoons water
artificial sweetener = 8 teaspoons sugar
½ teaspoon cinnamon

In a saucepan combine all the above ingredients and stir. Cover
and simmer very slowly. Make sure fruit is soft. Fill crêpes
with filling.

COFFEE SOUFFLÉ

Fiber per serving	0.15	¾ tablespoon unflavored gelatin
C/F	25.0	¾ cup strong cold coffee, di-
Rating	**M, R**	vided in half

¾ tablespoon unflavored gelatin
¾ cup strong cold coffee, divided in half
½ cup skim milk
1 heaping teaspoon bran
1 egg, separated
pinch salt
⅛ teaspoon vanilla
dietetic sweetener = 4 tablespoons sugar

In a bowl, soften the gelatin in half of the coffee and set aside. In the top of a double boiler, add the other half of the coffee, the milk, and the bran. Beat the egg yolk with the salt and then add it to the coffee mixture. Cook and stir until mixture starts to thicken. Add the gelatin and coffee mixture and cook a few more minutes, to make sure gelatin is completely dissolved. Remove double boiler from heat and add the vanilla and sweetener. Chill until it is thickened slightly. Beat the egg whites until they are very stiff and fold them in. Place entire mixture into individual dessert cups and chill until firm.

STRAWBERRIES AND CREAM

Fiber per serving	0.2	2 ounces cottage cheese
C/F	8.3	2 tablespoons skim milk
Rating	**M, R**	liquid or granulated dietetic

2 ounces cottage cheese
2 tablespoons skim milk
liquid or granulated dietetic sweetener = 1 teaspoon sugar
¼ cup canned strawberries, unsweetened

Put all ingredients in blender, reserving a few strawberries. Mix well for about 30 seconds. Pour into dessert dishes. Put extra strawberries on top.

ORANGE AND BANANA DELIGHT

Fiber per serving	**1.8**	
C/F	**23.0**	
Rating	**M, R**	

2   medium oranges, peeled and sectioned
1   medium banana, peeled and cut into 1-inch pieces
¼   cup orange juice
1   tablespoon dietetic cherry flavoring
1   heaping tablespoon fine bran
½   teaspoon sesame seeds

In a small bowl combine orange sections, banana pieces, orange juice, dietetic cherry flavoring, and bran. Mix them together well. Cover bowl with a piece of aluminum foil and chill in refrigerator until ready to use. When ready to serve, place sesame seeds on a small piece of aluminum foil and bake in a hot oven for about 2 minutes, until seeds are slightly browned. Divide refrigerated fruit mixture into 2 glasses. Sprinkle toasted sesame seeds over the fruit-filled glasses.

CHEESE-BANANA PIE

Crust

Fiber per serving	**1.5**	
C/F	**25.0**	
Rating	**M, R**	

2   slices whole wheat bread, made into bread crumbs (see p. 230)
¼   teaspoon cinnamon dietetic sweetener = ½ teaspoon sugar
1   heaping teaspoon fine bran

Combine all the ingredients and press firmly into small pie pan. Let harden.

Filling

1/4 teaspoon lemon juice
1/4 teaspoon almond extract
4 tablespoons water
2 envelopes unflavored gelatin
  dietetic sweetener = 3 teaspoons sugar
2 small ripe bananas, peeled
4 ounces farmer cheese
1/2 cup skim milk
1 heaping teaspoon fine bran

Combine lemon juice, almond extract, and water in a small saucepan. Add gelatin and dissolve over medium heat. Do not boil. Remove from heat and pour into a blender. Add the rest of the ingredients to the softened gelatin liquid. Blend until smooth and creamy. Pour this mixture into pie shell. Refrigerate for 1 hour.

PIE CRUST
(1 crust size)

Fiber per serving	1.1	1/2 cup whole wheat flour
C/F	23.0	2 tablespoons oil
Rating	M	1 tablespoon ice water
		1 heaping teaspoon fine bran
		1/4 teaspoon salt

Combine all ingredients in a bowl. Mix with a fork. Knead mixture until pastry can be formed into a ball. Hand-flatten dough and wrap it in wax paper. Place in refrigerator for about 2 hours. When thoroughly chilled, roll dough out on board. Place in an 8-inch pie pan. (Double recipe for 2 crust pies.)

FRUIT DRINK

Fiber per serving	1.6
C/F	8.4
Rating	**M, R**

1 cup unsweetened strawberries with juice, frozen or
canned
2 heaping tablespoons fine
bran
10 ice cubes
dietetic sweetener = 12 teaspoons sugar
½ cup skim milk

Place all ingredients in a blender and mix at high speed for 1
minute, until strawberries are dissolved.

COOKIES

SESAME COOKIES

Fiber per serving	1.5
C/F	17.0
Rating	**M**

¼ cup sesame seeds
¼ cup whole wheat flour
2 heaping teaspoons fine bran
dietetic brown sugar sweetener = 3 teaspoons brown
sugar
2 tablespoons raisins
¼ teaspoon coconut extract
¼ teaspoon vanilla extract
2 tablespoons oil
½ egg, beaten
pinch of salt

In a mixing bowl combine all ingredients and mix with a fork.
Make balls of cookie mixture with a tablespoon. Pat lightly. Put
on ungreased cookie sheet and flatten balls with back of a

spoon. Bake for about 20 minutes in a preheated 350° oven. Let cookies cool, then remove with a spatula. Can be frozen.

POPPY SEED COOKIES

Fiber per serving	1.5
C/F	17.0
Rating	**M**

¼ cup poppy seeds
3 heaping teaspoons bran
½ cup whole wheat flour
dietetic brown sugar sweetener =6 teaspoons brown
sugar
½ teaspoon almond extract
½ teaspoon vanilla extract
⅓ cup oil
1 egg
pinch of salt

Put all the ingredients in a mixing bowl. Mix well with a fork. Form the mixture into small balls. Do not roll. Place on an ungreased cookie sheet and press cookies down with a spoon to flatten them. Bake in a 350° oven (not preheated) for about 25 minutes until cookies are browned. Allow cookies to cool, then remove with spatula. Make cookies thin as they will be very crunchy. Can be frozen.

SNACKS

CRACKER CREATIONS I

Fiber per serving	0.7
C/F	18.0
Rating	**M, R**

6 Triscuit crackers
1 slice Swiss cheese, cut into 6
cracker-sized squares
½ medium tomato, sliced

½ medium tomato, sliced
1 tablespoon onion, diced
1 heaping teaspoon bran
1 tablespoon sesame seeds

On each cracker place a small piece of cheese and a slice of tomato. Sprinkle on onion, bran, and sesame seeds. Place crackers on a piece of aluminum foil and broil for about 5 minutes, or until cheese melts.

CRACKER CREATIONS II

Fiber per serving	**0.7**	6 Triscuit crackers
C/F	**16.0**	2 pieces American cheese, cut
Rating	**M, R**	in 6 cracker-sized squares
		1 tablespoon sesame seeds
		1 heaping teaspoon fine bran

On each cracker put a small piece of cheese and sprinkle with sesame seeds and bran. Place crackers on a piece of aluminum foil. Broil for about 3 minutes, or until cheese melts.

STUFFED MUSHROOMS

Fiber per serving	**0.8**	¼ pound whole fresh mushrooms, raw
C/F	**6.0**	2 ounces cheddar cheese, grated
Rating	**M, R**	1 heaping teaspoon fine bran
		½ teaspoon dried parsley, chopped
		½ tablespoon onion, minced
		2 small cloves garlic, chopped
		salt and pepper to taste
		1 teaspoon prepared mustard

Preheat oven to 375°. Wash and dry mushrooms. Remove stems of mushrooms and finely chop the mushroom stems. Add the cheddar cheese, bran, parsley, onion, and garlic. Add salt and pepper to taste. Then add the mustard and mix very well. Place mushroom caps with open side up on a cookie sheet. Spoon chopped mixture in each cap, in proportion to the size of the mushroom. Place in oven and bake for 15 to 20 minutes. Serve hot.

PIZZA

Fiber per serving	**1.3**	2 slices whole wheat bread
C/F	**12.0**	½ medium tomato, sliced
Rating	**M, R**	3 ounces skim milk mozzarella cheese, sliced
		⅛ pound fresh mushrooms, cut thin, or ½ can (2 ounces) sliced mushrooms, drained garlic powder, to taste oregano, to taste
		1 tablespoon bran

On each piece of bread place slices of tomato. Add the cheese and top with pieces of mushroom. Sprinkle with garlic powder and oregano to taste. Sprinkle with bran. Place on a piece of aluminum foil and broil until cheese bubbles.

CLAM DIP

Fiber per serving	**0.5**	¼ cup cottage cheese
C/F	**4.9**	½ can (8 ounce) minced clams, drained
Rating	**M, R**	3 drops Worcestershire sauce
		½ tablespoon chives

salt and pepper to taste
½ *tablespoon sesame seeds or*
poppy seeds
1 *heaping tablespoon bran*

Put cottage cheese into blender and blend until smoothed to sour-cream consistency. Add clams and other ingredients. Mix well. Can be used with raw vegetables.

SAUCES

TARTAR SAUCE

Fiber per serving	0.9
C/F	6.8
Rating	M

1 *heaping teaspoon fine bran*
1 *teaspoon prepared mustard*
2 *tablespoons pickle, chopped*
2 *tablespoons parsley, chopped*
1 *cup Mayonnaise Special*
(see next recipe)

Mix all ingredients together. Serve with fish.

MAYONNAISE SPECIAL
(yields 2½ cups)

Fiber per serving	
(depends on quantity)	
C/F	8.7
Rating	M

2 *egg yolks*
¼ *cup lemon juice*
2 *teaspoons prepared mustard*
1 *teaspoon salt*
artificial sweetener = 2 table-
spoons sugar
pinch of pepper
pinch of curry or cayenne
powder (optional)
1 *tablespoon fine bran*
2 *cups oil*

In a small bowl combine egg yolks, 2 teaspoons lemon juice, mustard, salt, sweetener, pepper, curry or cayenne powder, and bran. Mix well. Beat with electric mixer until mixture is thick. Add oil, drop by drop, and beat continuously. Add the rest of lemon juice. Place in refrigerator.

For variations add a few drops Worcestershire sauce or chopped chives.

NATURAL GRAVY

Fiber per serving	0.6	*1 cup natural gravy*
C/F	4.4	*1 heaping tablespoon fine bran*
Rating	**M, R**	

Add to natural gravy 1 tablespoon fine bran. Heat and serve.

RED PIMIENTO SAUCE

Fiber per serving	0.9	*1 can (7 ounces) pimientos,*
C/F	7.1	*drained*
Rating	**M, R**	*2 tablespoons vinegar*
		2 tablespoons prepared mustard
		1 heaping teaspoon fine bran dietetic sweetener =4 teaspoons sugar

In a blender combine all ingredients. Blend until smooth. Chill in refrigerator. Use over Tacos (see p. 167).

RED HOT SAUCE
(for broiled fish)

Fiber per serving	0.3	*2 tablespoons vinegar*
C/F	15.0	*¼ cup water*
Rating	**M, R**	*2 tablespoons ketchup*

½ tablespoon prepared mustard
dash of Tabasco sauce
dietetic sweetener = 1½ teaspoons sugar
½ tablespoon parsley, chopped
dash lemon-pepper marinade
1 heaping teaspoon bran

In a small saucepan place all the above ingredients. Stir well
and cook on low heat for 10 minutes. Spoon over broiled fish
before serving.

RED CREOLE SAUCE
(for fish)

Fiber per serving	2.7	
C/F	6.2	
Rating	**M, R**	

1 can (8 ounces) tomato sauce
½ cup water
½ medium cucumber, peeled
and diced
½ medium green pepper,
diced
1½ tablespoons parsley flakes,
minced
1 tablespoon dehydrated
onion flakes
½ stalk celery, finely diced
½ clove garlic
¼ cup water
¼ cup clam juice
1 tablespoon instant chicken
broth
1 tablespoon fine bran
½ teaspoon salt
dash of pepper

In a saucepan cook tomato sauce and water until the liquid is reduced by half. Add all the remaining ingredients. Boil and then let mixture simmer for about 15 minutes. Be sure vegetables are crisp yet tender. Serve over baked fish.

BREAD CRUMBS
(to use for pie crusts, stuffing, or in other recipes)

Fiber per serving	1.0	
C/F	12.8	
Rating	depends on quantity	

2 slices whole wheat bread, 2 or 3 days old, or lightly toasted

2 heaping teaspoons fine bran seasonings or spices to taste

Take 2 slices of whole wheat bread that is at least 2 or 3 days old and put into blender. If bread is fresh toast it lightly. Add 2 heaping teaspoons fine bran, and any seasonings or spices you desire. Blend for about 30 seconds, until bread is well crumbed.

SYRUP

Fiber per serving	0.5	
C/F	14.0	
Rating	M, R	

¼ cup dietetic jelly, any flavor

¼ cup water

¾ tablespoon whole wheat flour

1 heaping teaspoon fine bran

In a saucepan combine the jelly and the water. Cook until the jelly dissolves. Then add the flour and bran. Cook until the mixture thickens, stirring constantly. Refrigerate. Use over whole wheat pancakes.

HONEY DIETETIC
SWEETENER COMBO

For those who want the flavor of honey, but not all the calories, I suggest a mixture of honey and dietetic sweetener. To each teaspoon of honey add in drops of liquid dietetic sweetener the equivalent of two teaspoons sugar. One teaspoon of this combination is equal in sweetness to three teaspoons of honey.

CHAPTER 12

CARBOHYDRATE-FIBER
TABLES

Tables like these have never been published for the general public before, for two reasons. First, the carbohydrate-fiber ratio is a brand-new concept. Second, the importance of fiber in the diet is just being recognized for the first time. These new tables may give you some of the information you need to be successful in losing weight and in controlling your weight.

These tables differ in five ways from almost all of the tables that are commonly available. From my experience in this field, I can tell you that these are valuable improvements.

1. *Carbohydrate-fiber ratio.* This new concept tells you the value of foods that grow from the ground, or that are made from plant foods. The detailed explanation of the carbohydrate-fiber ratio, including the formula by which it is calculated, is found in Chapter 5.

The C/F is the best guide available to how "naked" are the calories you eat. When you choose between foods to eat, particularly on The High-Fiber Reducing Diet, you should strive to eat the foods with the lowest C/F.

2. *Fiber.* The amount of fiber in food is often impossible to find in common calorie tables. Yet you need to know this if you are to determine the total amount of fiber in your daily diet.

3. *Carbohydrate.* Unlike the usual carbohydrate values given in tables, these tables contain only "available" carbo-

hydrates. The amounts of indigestible carbohydrate have already been subtracted.

4. *Calories.* Many of these calorie values are also different from previous tables you have seen. This is the result of subtracting the calories of those carbohydrates that are unavailable to you.

5. *Ratings.* I have prepared ratings that tell you how good each food is for dieting, for weight control, and for good health, according to its C/F and the number of calories it contains. The following code is used in the rating column:

Rating	Explanation
M	Acceptable on The Weight-Maintenance Diet.
N	Conditionally acceptable on The Weight-Maintenance Diet if the C/F is lowered by adding additional fiber.
R	Acceptable on The High-Fiber Reducing Diet.
S	Conditionally acceptable on The High-Fiber Reducing Diet if the C/F is lowered by adding fiber.
T	Acceptable on The High-Fiber Reducing Diet in limited quantities.
X	Unacceptable as a healthy food because of the naked calories in the form of sugar.
Y	Unacceptable as a healthy food because of the naked calories in the form of other refined carbohydrates.

These five changes, the C/F, the amount of fiber, omitting "unavailable" carbohydrates, listing only "available" calories, and the new rating system, make these tables more desirable for dieters than most of the others that I have seen.

OTHER REMARKS

Fruits and vegetables. Unless otherwise stated, the figures are given for fruits and vegetables in the raw state. Values are only for the edible portions. Unless stated otherwise, they are fresh rather than canned.

Unusually large C/F numbers. When the amount of fiber is so small that it is only a trace (or none is present at all), then the C/F becomes unusually large. It is then designated with the infinity sign (∞). This sign means that these foods are unacceptable.

Accuracy. Every attempt has been made to achieve accuracy in these tables, but complete accuracy is impossible since foods vary in composition from one locale to another and from one season to another. You should consider tabulated data such as this as a general approximation.

Absolute accuracy is not even required, since these values are meant to serve you only as a guide. Sometimes, where exact information is not available, I have done my best to give you the information by careful estimation from the information that is available.

C/F TABLES

Food (100 gms)	C/F	Fiber	Carbo-hydrate	Calories	Rating
Almonds ⅔ cup	6.3	2.7	17.0	536	M
Apples 1 small, 2 inch	14.0	1.0	14.0	54	M, R
Applesauce canned, sweetened ⅓ cup	46.0	0.5	23.0	89	X
Applesauce canned, unsweetened ½ cup	17.0	0.6	10.0	41	M, R
Apricots 2 medium	20.0	0.6	12.0	49	M, R
Artichokes ½ large	3.4	2.4	8.2	69	M, T

C / F TABLES—Continued

Food (100 gms)	C/F	Fiber	Carbo-hydrate	Calories	Rating
Asparagus 6 spears	6.1	0.7	4.3	23	M, R
Avocados ½ fruit	2.9	1.6	4.7	161	M, T
Bananas 1 small	44.0	0.5	22.0	83	M, S
Beans, dry, white ½ cup	13.0	4.3	57.0	323	M, T
Beans, Lima, dry ½ cup	14.0	4.3	60.0	328	M, T
Beans, Mung, dry 3½ ounces	13.0	4.4	56.0	323	M, T
Beans, Snap, Green 1 cup	6.1	1.0	6.1	28	M, R
Beets, red 2 beets	11.0	0.8	9.1	40	M, R
Blackberries ⅝ cup	2.15	4.1	8.8	42	M, R
Blueberries ⅝ cup	9.2	1.5	13.8	56	M, R
Bran Cereal, packaged 2½ cups	30.0	2.3	68.0	307	X
Bran Flakes, 40% packaged cereal 2½ cups	75.0	1.0	75.0	343	X
Bran Flakes, unprocessed *	4.4	12.0	53.0	312	M, R
Brazil Nuts ⅓ cup	4.2	2.1	8.9	638	M
Bread, Whole Wheat 4 slices	26.0	1.8	46.0	235	M, T
Broccoli 1 stalk	2.9	1.5	4.4	26	M, R
Brussels Sprouts 3½ ounces	4.0	1.6	6.7	39	M, R

* These are approximations based on best information available.

C/F TABLES—*Continued*

Food (100 gms)	C/F	Fiber	Carbo-hydrate	Calories	Rating
Buckwheat Groats ½ cup	44.0	1.6	70.0	347	M, S
Bun, Hamburger 3 buns	177.0	0.3	53.0	297	X, Y
Cabbage 1 cup shredded	5.8	0.8	4.6	21	M, R
Cake, Chocolate (Devil's Food) 1 piece without icing	260.0	0.2	52.0	367	X, Y
Cake, Devil's Food (from mix) 3½ ounces	257.0	0.3	77.0	406	X, Y
Cake, Pound 1 piece	∞	tr.	47.0	473	X, Y
Cake, Sponge 1 piece without icing	∞	0.0	54.0	298	X, Y
Cake, Yellow, mix, dry 3½ ounces	775.0	0.1	77.5	438	X, Y
Cantaloupe ¼ melon	24.0	0.3	7.2	29	M, R
Carrots 1 large	8.7	1.0	8.7	38	M, R
Cashew Nuts, roasted 1 cup	20.0	1.4	28.0	555	M
Catsup 3 ounces	50.0	0.5	25.0	104	N
Cauliflower 1 cup	4.2	1.0	4.2	23	M, R
Celery 1 cup diced	5.5	0.6	3.3	15	M, R
Cherries 12–15 large	43.0	0.4	17.0	68	M, S
Cherries, canned in syrup ½ cup	230.0	0.1	23.0	89	X

C/F TABLES—*Continued*

Food (100 gms)	C/F	Fiber	Carbo-hydrate	Calories	Rating
Chickpeas (Garbanzos) ½ cup dried	11.0	5.0	56.0	340	M, T
Coconut, fresh, shredded 1 cup	2.9	3.3	9.5	338	M
Cookies, Sugar Wafers 2 wafers	∞	tr.	73.0	482	X, Y
Cookies, Vanilla Wafers 3 wafers	∞	tr.	75.0	464	X, Y
Corn, Sweet 1 medium ear	30.0	0.7	21.0	93	M
Corn Flakes, dry 4 cups	104.0	0.8	83.0	376	X
Corn Meal, yellow, dry ¾ cup	133.0	0.6	80.0	372	N
Cornbread Mix, dry 3½ ounces	237.0	0.3	71.0	431	Y
Cranberry Sauce, canned 5 tablespoons	185.0	0.2	37.0	145	X
Cream of Wheat 2½ cups cooked	247.0	0.3	74.0	350	Y
Cucumbers 1 medium	4.7	0.6	2.8	14	M, R
Danish Pastry 3 small	153.0	0.3	46.0	423	X, Y
Dates, dried ⅝ cup	32.0	2.3	73.0	265	N
Doughnut—cake type, plain 3 doughnuts	∞	tr.	51.0	391	X, Y
Eclair, custard filling 1 average	∞	0.0	36.0	287	X, Y
Eggplant 2 slices	5.4	0.9	4.9	21	M, R
Figs, dried ⅔ cup	11.4	5.6	64.0	252	M

C/F TABLES—*Continued*

Food (100 gms)	C/F	Fiber	Carbo-hydrate	Calories	Rating
Flour, Buckwheat, dark *1 cup*	44.0	1.6	70.4	327	M, S
Flour, Cornmeal, ground *⁴/₅ cup*	79.0	0.9	71.0	343	N
Flour, Rye, medium dark *3½ ounces*	74.0	1.0	74.0	346	N
Flour, Soy *1⅓ cups*	12.0	2.4	28.0	411	M, S
Flour, Soy, defatted *¾ cup*	16.0	2.3	36.0	317	M, S
Flour, Wheat Gluten *⅔ cup*	10.0	3.8	40.0	340	M, T
Flour, White, All purpose *⅞ cup*	253.0	0.3	76.0	364	Y
Flour, Whole Wheat *¾ cup*	30.0	2.3	69.0	325	M, S
Fruit Cocktail, *canned, syrup* *½ cup*	48.0	0.4	19.0	74	X
Grapefruit, white *½ medium*	55.0	0.2	11.0	40	M
Grapes *20–30 grapes*	25.0	0.6	15.0	67	M, T
Honey *5 tablespoons*	780.0	0.1	78.0	306	X
Honeydew Melon *¼ small*	12.0	0.6	7.1	31	M, R
Icing, Chocolate, *frozen* *1 piece*	86.0	0.7	60.0	417	X
Jams *3½ ounces*	117.0	0.6	70.0	276	X
Jellies *3½ ounces*	∞	0.0	65.0	252	X
Juice, Apple—canned *²/₅ cup*	120.0	0.1	12.0	47	N

C/F TABLES—*Continued*

Food (100 gms)	C/F	Fiber	Carbo-hydrate	Calories	Rating
Juice, Grape—bottled 2/5 cup	∞	tr.	17.0	66	N
Juice, Grapefruit— fresh 2/5 cup	∞	tr.	9.2	39	N
Juice, Orange—fresh 2/5 cup	100.0	0.1	10.0	45	N
Juice, Pineapple— canned 2/5 cup	130.0	0.1	13.0	55	N
Juice, Prune—canned 2/5 cup	∞	tr.	19.0	77	N
Juice, Tomato—canned 2/5 cup	21.0	0.2	4.1	18	M, R
Lemons 1 lemon	20.0	0.4	7.8	25	M, R
Lettuce, Iceberg 3½ ounces	4.0	0.5	2.0	12	M, R
Mangos ½ medium	18.0	0.9	16.0	62	M, T
Molasses, Blackstrap 5 tablespoons	∞	0.0	55.0	213	X
Mushrooms 10 small	4.5	0.8	3.6	25	M, R
Oatmeal 2½ cups	45.0	1.5	68.0	356	M, S
Okra 3½ ounces	6.6	1.0	6.6	32	M, R
Onions 1 onion	14.0	0.6	8.1	36	M, R
Onions (Scallions) 5 onions	9.5	1.0	9.5	41	M, R
Oranges 1 small	24.0	0.5	12.0	47	M, R

C/F TABLES—*Continued*

Food (100 gms)	C/F	Fiber	Carbo-hydrate	Calories	Rating
Pancakes 1 average (5½ inch diameter)	160.0	0.2	32.0	231	X, Y
Peaches 1 medium	15.0	0.6	9.1	36	M, R
Peaches, canned in syrup 2 halves	50.0	0.4	20.0	76	X
Peaches, canned in juice 2 halves	28.0	0.4	11.0	43	M, T
Peanut Butter 6 to 7 tablespoons	9.5	2.0	19.0	568	M, X *
Peanuts, roasted without skin 3½ ounces	11.0	1.5	17.0	560	M
Pears ½ fruit	10.0	1.4	14.0	55	M, T
Pears, canned, in juice ²/₅ cup	11.0	0.7	8.0	29	M, R
Pears, canned, in syrup 2 halves	32.0	0.6	19.0	74	X
Pear Nectar, canned 3 ounces	43.0	0.3	13.0	51	X
Peas, Green ¾ cup shelled	6.0	2.0	12.0	76	M, T
Peppers, Green 1 large	2.4	1.4	3.4	16	M, R
Pickles, Dill 1 large	3.4	0.5	1.7	9	M, R
Pie, Apple 1 small slice	95.0	0.4	38.0	254	X, Y
Pie, Blueberry ¹/₁₀ pie	49.0	0.7	34.0	239	X, Y

* Depends on brand. Those with sugar are rated X.

C/F TABLES—Continued

Food (100 gms)	C/F	Fiber	Carbo-hydrate	Calories	Rating
Pie, Lemon Meringue 1/8 pie	∞	tr.	38.0	255	X, Y
Pineapple 3/4 cup	33.0	0.4	13.0	52	M
Pineapple, canned, in syrup 1 large slice with syrup	63.0	0.3	19.0	74	X
Pineapple, canned, in juice 1 slice with juice	50.0	0.3	15.0	58	N
Pistachio Nuts 50 nuts	8.5	2.0	17.0	580	M
Plums 2 medium	43.0	0.4	17.0	64	M
Potatoes, white 1 medium	34.0	0.5	17.0	76	M
Prunes, dried 10–15 prunes	41.0	1.6	66.0	249	N
Radishes, Red 10 radishes	4.0	0.7	2.9	14	M, R
Raisins, dried seedless 3½ ounces	76.0	1.0	76.0	286	N
Ralston 2⅓ cups cooked	33.0	2.1	70.0	329	M, S
Raspberries, Red 3/4 cup	3.7	3.0	11.0	45	M, R
Rhubarb 3½ ounces	17.0	0.7	3.0	13	M, R
Rice, brown 2⅓ cups cooked	101.0	0.7	71.0	361	N
Rice, brown, dry ½ cup	95.0	0.8	77.0	355	N
Rice, white 2⅓ cups	200.0	0.4	80.0	368	Y
Rice, white, dry ½ cup	400.0	0.2	80.0	363	Y

C/F TABLES—*Continued*

Food (100 gms)	C/F	Fiber	Carbo-hydrate	Calories	Rating
Sauerkraut, canned ⅔ cup	4.7	0.7	3.3	15	M, R
Soup, Chicken Noodle, canned ½ serving	34.0	0.1	3.4	25	N
Soup, Chicken Vegetable ⅖ cup	39.0	0.1	3.9	30	M, S
Soup, Clam Chowder ⅖ cup	20.0	0.2	4.0	30	M, S
Soup, Creamed Chicken with milk ⅖ cup	54.0	0.1	5.4	73	N
Soup, Green Pea, canned ½ serving	10.0	0.8	8.0	52	N, S
Soup, Onion ⅖ cup	9.0	0.2	1.8	26	M, S
Soup, Tomato ⅖ cup	20.0	0.3	5.9	36	M, S
Soup, Vegetable Beef ⅖ cup	9.3	0.3	2.8	30	M, S
Spinach 3½ ounces	6.0	0.6	3.7	24	M, R
Squash, Summer ½ cup	6.0	0.6	3.6	17	M, R
Strawberries 10 large	5.5	1.3	7.1	32	M, R
Strawberries, frozen 3½ ounces	38.0	0.6	23.0	91	M
Sugar, brown, crude 7 tablespoons	910.0	0.1	91.0	356	X
Sugar, white, table ½ cup	∞	0.0	99.5	385	X
Sunflower Seed kernels 3½ ounces	4.2	3.8	16.0	545	M
Sweet Potatoes 1 small	37.0	0.7	26.0	111	M

244

C/F TABLES—*Continued*

Food (100 gms)	C/F	Fiber	Carbo-hydrate	Calories	Rating
Tangerine 1 large	22.0	0.5	11.0	44	M, R
Tomato 1 small	8.4	0.5	4.2	20	M, R
Tomato Paste—canned 3½ ounces	20.0	0.9	18.0	78	M, T
Turnip Greens ½ cup	5.3	0.8	4.2	25	M, R
Waffles 1 waffle (7½ inch diameter)	370.0	0.1	37.0	279	X, Y
Walnuts, English 1 cup	6.7	2.1	14.0	648	M
Water Chestnuts, Chinese 3½ ounces	23.0	0.8	18.0	75	M, T
Watermelon, ripe	20.0	0.3	6.1	25	M, R
Wheat, shredded	35.0	2.3	81.0	372	M, S
Wheat Germ 3½ ounces	18.0	2.5	44.2	353	M, T
Wheatena 2⅓ cups	42.0	1.8	76.0	354	N
Wild Rice ⅞ cup	67.0	1.1	74.0	350	N

CHAPTER **13**

FOOD RESOURCES AND CONSUMER ADVICE

There are many products on the market, found in both health-food stores and in supermarkets, that fulfill the recommendations made in this book. This list is by no means complete. It simply shows a number of easily found products that I happen to like. I'm sure there are many that perhaps are not available in my particular area, but that are just as good or even better. Use this list as a guide to the types of products which are available, but certainly not as an emphatic mandate to buy only the products mentioned.

EGG SUBSTITUTES

Second Nature: This is about the only egg substitute that I have found that is low calorie. It is quite acceptable alone or as a substitute for eggs in cooking. Rating M, R.

CRACKERS

Ry-King: Swedish Crisp Bread (Golden Rye, Light Rye, and Brown Rye). A satisfactory cracker. Rating M.
Finn-Crisp: A satisfactory cracker. Rating M.
Triscuit: A satisfactory cracker. Rating M.

CEREALS

Uncle Sam Cereal: Satisfactory. Rating M, R.
Ralston Cereal: Good hot cereal. Rating M, R.
Wheatena: Good hot cereal. Rating M, R.
Good Shepherd Almonds 'n Molasses Cereal: Usually found in health-food stores. Rating M, S.
Roman Meal Cereals: Probably found only in health-food stores. Rating M, T.
Elam's 100% Whole Cracked Wheat Cereal: A hot cereal. Rating A, T.
Grape-Nuts: An excellent cereal, but not *Grape-Nuts Flakes,* which contain sugar. Rating M, R.
Shredded Wheat: Any brand. Available also in bite size. Rating M, T.

RICE

Brown Rice: Any brand of unprocessed brown rice is acceptable on The Weight-Maintenance Diet.

CHEESE

There are a number of low calorie cheese products.
Di-et Cheese: A low-calorie cheese product. Rating M, R.
Count Down: A low-calorie cheese spread. Rating M, R.
Life-line Neufchatel Cheese: A low-calorie cheese. Rating M, R.
Part-Skim-Milk Mozzarella Cheese: Rating M, T.
Jarlsberg Cheese: A part-skim-milk cheese with Swiss cheese-like flavor, but from Norway. Rating M, T.
Low Fat Cottage Cheese: There are a number of brands available. Two that I usually prefer are *Stay 'n Shape* and *Light 'n Lively.* Rating M, R.

CANNED FRUIT

Most fruits canned without added sugar or honey are acceptable, but for specific ratings see the tables.

Mott's Apple Sauce (without sugar): One of several sugarless apple sauces. Rating M, R.

FLAVORINGS AND SEASONINGS

Virtually any spice or seasoning is acceptable, although watch out for sauces that contain sugar.
Marmite, Savorex, Vegex: Meaty flavorings made from yeast extract. Some are found only in health-food stores. Rating M, R.

MILK

Whole Milk: May be used on The Weight-Maintenance Diet, but certainly not to excess.
Skim Milk: Should be used on The High-Fiber Reducing Diet when you consume milk.
Nonfat Dry Milk: Many available brands. Rating M, T.

FRYING AIDS

Cooking Oil: May be used to fry food on The Weight-Maintenance Diet.
Vegetable Sprays: On The High-Fiber Reducing Diet use any of the nonstick skillet sprays. There are several on the market, and they are all satisfactory.

BEVERAGES

The key, of course, is no refined carbohydrates or sugar. Therefore, diet sodas are encouraged and virtually all of them are acceptable on both The Weight-Maintenance Diet and The High-Fiber Reducing Diet.

An Explanation of Epidemiological Evidence with Mythical Examples

The most striking new information this book offers comes from epidemiological evidence. Indeed, many of the greatest breakthroughs in the history of medicine were sparked by this kind of evidence.

So that you can judge the message of this book, I will give you a quick understanding of epidemiological evidence. Two imaginary examples will explain it.

Suppose a laboratory researcher hypothesizes that many people are below average height because they suffered a deficiency of a certain growth factor in their diet during childhood. He calls it growth factor X. He knows that the growth factor is present in a number of different foods, but one good source is bananas.

To test his hypothesis in the laboratory, he designs an experiment in which he takes 200 white mice, all approximately one month of age, and separates them into two groups. Group A is fed a diet that excludes any food that he believes contains growth factor X. Group B is fed the exact same foods with the exception that bananas are added daily. He meticulously measures the length of each mouse at the onset of the experiment and at regular intervals during it.

At the end of several months he records the data, makes calculations, and discovers that the average length of the mice in Group B is one and one half inches longer than the average length in Group A. He therefore comes to the conclusion that growth factor X is responsible for this difference. These conclusions will be set forth in a scientific paper describing his experiment, and will be known as experimental evidence.

This evidence will have to be evaluated for exactly what it does and does not prove. For one thing, it does not say that growth factor X has any effect on the growth of humans, since the subjects of the experiment were mice. Secondly, it does not even prove that growth factor X is the reason for the increased growth in the mice in Group B, since the mice were fed bananas and the increased growth could have been produced by other factors in the bananas. But it is evident that some factor in the bananas caused the difference, and in later experiments, the researcher will probably attempt to chemically isolate growth factor X and use it alone instead of bananas.

Before the hypothesis could become medically accepted for people, the researcher will have to do a safe, carefully designed experiment on human subjects, and since humans grow proportionately much slower than mice, this would take at least several years.

Now let us look at epidemiological evidence. This comes directly from the real world, not the laboratory. Suppose in Cornville, Iowa, a city with a population of 250,000 people, a manufacturing plant is built to produce a new, super-hard plastic, called Z-plastic. This is to be the first plant of its kind in the world. The site for the plant is chosen because the raw material for this plastic is corn and corn husks, and this raw material is abundant in Iowa.

The city government is very pleased to bring this new industry to Cornville, though a number of ecologically minded people are up in arms over the threat of air pollution. Nonetheless, the plant is completed with the usual, loudly trumpeted public relations assurances that the smoke rising from the smokestacks will be well filtered to remove harmful ingredients.

Within a year doctors and hospitals in Cornville report an alarming increase in bronchitis and pneumonia, as well as a rising number of deaths from pneumonia. Small towns within a short distance from Cornville, and those farther away but downwind from it, also report an increased incidence of these ailments, but to a lesser extent.

In addition, after the plant has been in operation for a year, physicians and dermatologists note that they are seeing an increased number of patients whose complaint is falling hair and baldness. Many of these patients are women.

The most distressing change, however, is an increased incidence of hepitoma, or cancer of the liver. Many new cases are noted and the number of cases per thousand population is steadily rising far above its formerly low level, and is climbing above any other area in the United States.

To continue with our mythical tragedy, the Russians, not wanting to be left behind, build twice as large a Z-plastic plant in the city of Kiev, in the corn-rich area of the Ukraine. Lo and behold, they too begin to show an increased incidence of lung diseases, death from pneumonia, baldness, and cancer of the liver.

Back in Cornville, an aggressive young newspaper reporter was interviewing a doctor on another story, and got wind of these new diseases. He dug out the facts, and wrote a hardhitting series of articles. National attention resulted and local environmentalists began a long, slow battle to close the plant. There was a change of administration in Washington after the next presidential election, and the new head of the Environmental Protection Agency was ordered to review the case. The EPA decided to join the fight and the plastics plant was closed by court order, four and a half years after it opened. Within a year after the closing the number of cases of bronchitis and pneumonia decreased to normal levels, as did the baldness. During the same period the number of cases of cancer of the liver fell to the same rate as the rest of the population of the United States, even though the city had had a lower rate of hepitoma before.

Unfortunately, a class-action lawsuit to recover damages was stalled in the courts for years. Because the courts placed expensive notification requirements on those who brought the suit, they were eventually forced to drop the suit when their fund-raising drive fell short of its goal. To the very end, their lawyers assured them they were entitled to damages for what they had suffered as innocent victims. But because of expensive court ordered notification requirements, not a dime of compensation was ever paid.

At the same time several laboratory researchers subjected a number of groups of mice to various chemicals found in the smoke emitted from the Z-plastic plant. Unfortunately, the results were inconclusive. Some mice developed lung ailments, but many didn't. Several mice shed great quantities of hair, but none became bald or hairless. Other mice developed diseases completely unrelated to any the citizens of Cornville encountered. There was a great deal of discussion among these scientists as to why the experiments on mice produced these results. It was concluded that they produced no significant evidence that could be applied to the plight of the people of Cornville.

The evidence that the Z-plastic plant was responsible for the increase in the ailments suffered by some people in Cornville, probably through the smoke that was emitted, is called epidemiological evidence. It amounts to strong suspicions, based on the geographical location of the epidemic and subsidence of the symptoms once the causative agents are removed.

The epidemiological evidence was not 100 percent conclusive, but the fact that the ailments began with the opening of the plant and disappeared with the closing of the plant—and were present only in the area of the plant—was strong evidence that there was a relationship. The evidence was further supported by the similar findings reported from Russia, where the doctors reported their medical opinions only to the state authority and the international medical literature. Unfortunately, the state decided to keep their plant operating in spite of its hazards, and closed it after ten years only when the incidence of disease became intolerable.

Had the courts in America waited for the experimental evidence to prove the dangers from this air pollution, many of the people in the city would have died. Sometimes it is necessary to act immediately on the strength of this kind of evidence to save lives and to safeguard the public's health.

One of Cornville's doctors who had seen an abnormally large number of cases of baldness decided to name the condition Z-plastic baldness. Other doctors followed suit, calling different manifestations Z-plastic lung disease and Z-plastic cancer.

Statistically it was found that most of the people who suffered the effects of "plastic pollution" showed these effects only in one area, that is, they only had one of the three diseases. However, 40 percent of those who had pneumonia in Cornville during those years also experienced falling hair and patches of baldness. But only 1 percent of these people also contracted cancer of the liver.

Why some people did not contract any of these ailments, while others contracted one, two, or all three, was the subject of intense medical debate. It was concluded that different individuals had different inherent predispositions for each of the diseases.

Years later, the medical textbooks described what had occurred in Cornville and Kiev. They referred to it as one disease, the Z-plastic disease. The textbooks described three distinct manifestations of the disease: baldness, lung illness, and cancer. The textbooks could have listed three different diseases, but when one cause produces three diseases, it is medically recognized as one disease with three separate manifestations.

Z-plastic disease is an imaginary example, but what we have learned from it is very real. Based upon better evidence than in our example above, there is a disease epidemic that is rampant in America, in every city and town, practically in every house and apartment, from one end of our country to the other. In fact, it could be called a plague, because millions of people have died from it, and millions more have been stricken and forced to live diminished lives.

The cause of this real epidemic is not in Cornville, in a plastics factory. It is in the diets of almost all Americans. When you sit down to eat your very next meal, if you do not get sufficient fiber you may be furthering this epidemic, helping it strike in your home, helping it shorten your life. There is a great deal of epidemiological evidence that backs up this incredible statement.

How you can stop this epidemic in your own home, put up a dietary barricade and lock it out, is the subject of this book, but to make your campaign successful, you have to understand where this epidemic comes from. If you don't know why you should add fiber to your diet and eliminate refined carbohydrates, no authority can convince you to do it. If you do know why you should make this change, no public-relations campaign by any special interest will be able to stop you.

The Do-It-Yourself Transit Time Test

It would be very desirable for you to know just what your own transit time is. The test can be done rather simply in a laboratory, but it presents certain problems if it is attempted at home. If your doctor or a researcher performed this test on you, he or she would probably have you swallow some substance called a marker, a material that would show up on an X-ray film. The doctor would note the time at which you swallowed it and instruct you to note the times of your bowel movements. You would bring your stools to the doctor in a plastic bag, where they would be X-rayed. When the marker showed up on film, the doctor would calculate how long it took to pass through you. Sometimes these tests are done by having the subject swallow a dye. Various other materials have been used.

Since you cannot conveniently use X-rays at home, I must have you swallow something that will be easily recognizable in the toilet bowl and have you do your own timing. The most logical material would be some foodstuff that is not readily digestible, and which you could easily recognize when it appeared. I have tried various things, two of which seem acceptable.

One is millet seed, which is a tiny round seed available very inexpensively in health-food stores. Another is unpopped popcorn. One brand I particularly like is made by the Reese Company, and they call it Confetti. The kernels are brightly colored red, blue, green, orange, yellow, etc., although the color may be somewhat lost in transit, there is more chance of identifying this particular brand.

The procedure is as follows: Be sure that you have eaten no other corn within four days of doing the test, or the results might be confusing. Simply swallow, with water, 30 or 40 kernels of corn. Note the time. Each time you have a bowel movement for the next three or four days, look at the stool for evidence of the corn kernels. Here is where the problem lies. Some subjects on whom this test was done were not able to identify the corn.

If you prefer to use millet seeds, about 1 teaspoon of seed will do. The seeds will appear as somewhat yellowish polka dots in the stool.

The test should not be repeated more often than once every three or four weeks, and after you are stabilized on the right amount of bran, there should be little need to repeat the test. Your goal is a transit time ranging from twenty-four to thirty-six hours.

The Amount of Fiber in Bran

There seems to be some variation in what different sources and authorities report as the fiber content of bran. I have researched many sources, and as a result have decided to use the standard of 12 percent. I realize that particular batches of bran, depending on the type of wheat, the region in which it was grown, and the kind of milling procedure, may vary. For those who are interested in some research sources, I would recommend:

· Shetlar, M. R., Rankin, G. T., Lyman, J. F., and France, W. G. "Investigation of the Proximate Chemical Composition of the Separate Bran Layers of Wheat." *Cereal Chemistry,* Vol. 24, pp. 111–122, 1947.
· Kent-Jones, D. W. and Amos, A. J. *Modern Cereal Chemistry,* Chapters 1 and 8. Liverpool, England: The Northern Publishing Company, 1947.
· Pearson, David. *The Chemical Analysis of Foods,* Chapter 5. London, England: J. and A. Churchill, 1970.

The following tables indicate the lengths to which I went to determine the amount of bran that should be added to the diet as a supplement. I did this entire procedure several times, over a period of six months. Overall, I achieved approximately the same results in every trial. The following tables are included for two reasons. First, they illustrate the procedure which I followed, and second, they are near the midpoint of the range for all the trials, and thus have been used as the basis for my recommendations in the book.

I went to the housewares department of several department stores and purchased four different styles of measuring spoons. Two were plastic and two were metal. Then I used the same procedure to weigh the following measures of both bran and fine bran:

- · 1 level teaspoon
- · 1 "small heap" heaping teaspoon
- · 1 "largest heap possible" heaping teaspoon
- · 1 "small heap" heaping tablespoon
- · 1 "largest heap possible" heaping tablespoon

All of these measurements were done on a triple-beam chemical balance, which is accurate to one-tenth of a gram. Let me explain how I arrived at the measurement for the "small heap" heaping teaspoon; this will serve as an example of the other measurements that were made, because the procedure was the same.

First, a paper bowl was put on the chemical balance and weighed. It weighed 10.2 grams. Then I used a readily available bran product (my tests of various brands showed that different brands weigh almost exactly the same, for the same volume) and began with the first style measuring spoon, the stainless steel one. To get a "small heap" I took a large heaping teaspoonful, and shook the spoon lightly, knocking off the excess amount and leaving a nicely rounded pile. I took 10 of these teaspoonfuls and added them to the bowl on the chemical balance, weighed the entire amount, and subtracted the weight of the bowl. This gave the total weight of 10 teaspoonfuls, and I divided this by 10 to get the weight of one average teaspoon.

Next I did the same with the other three measuring spoons,

the round plastic, the oval plastic, and the round aluminum. I got the weight of an average "small heap" for each of them, then averaged them together to produce an average weight for the "small heap" teaspoonful.

To arrive at the figure I used in the book, I did the same series of measurements for the "largest heap possible" heaping teaspoon, and then used a figure between the two. In this way, when I recommend the use of "heaping" teaspoons and "heaping" tablespoons in the recipes, you should be taking an amount that is larger than the "small heap," but not so large that the slightest quiver will spill some of the bran. Just use the largest size heaping teaspoon or heaping tablespoon that is comfortable and quick, and you will be very close to the figure that I recommend and the weights that are given in Chapter 7.

The following tables point out just how complex this simple measurement can get. They include the measurements for both regular bran and for fine bran, in all of the styles of measuring spoons used for the teaspoon and the tablespoon. These tables should answer any questions you might have about where the measurements of bran come from.

TEASPOON REGULAR BRAN
LEVEL

(All weights in grams)	Stainless Steel	Round Plastic	Oval Plastic	Round Aluminum
Weight of container	10.2	10.2	10.2	10.2
Weight of container plus 10 level tsp. bran	19.1	20.8	20.0	19.9
Weight of 10 tsp. bran alone	8.9	10.6	9.8	9.7
Weight of one level tsp. bran	0.89	1.1	0.98	0.97

Mean weight of bran contained in one level teaspoon
of those tested: 0.99

TEASPOON REGULAR BRAN
HEAPING (SMALL HEAP)

(All weights in grams)	Stainless Steel	Round Plastic	Oval Plastic	Round Aluminum
Weight of container	*10.2*	*10.2*	*10.2*	*10.2*
Weight of container plus 10 heaping tsp. bran (small heap)	*28.7*	*26.5*	*29.3*	*30.7*
Weight of 10 tsp. bran alone	*18.5*	*16.3*	*19.1*	*20.5*
Weight of one heaping tsp. bran (small heap)	*1.9*	*1.6*	*1.9*	*2.1*

Mean weight of bran contained in one heaping teaspoon
(small heap) of those tested: 1.9

TEASPOON REGULAR BRAN
HEAPING (LARGEST HEAP POSSIBLE)

(All weights in grams)	Stainless Steel	Round Plastic	Oval Plastic	Round Aluminum
Weight of container	*10.2*	*10.2*	*10.2*	*10.2*
Weight of container plus 10 heaping tsp. bran (largest heap possible)	*33.8*	*30.6*	*34.0*	*35.6*
Weight of 10 tsp. bran alone	*23.6*	*20.4*	*23.8*	*25.4*
Weight of one heaping tsp. bran (largest heap possible)	*2.4*	*2.0*	*2.4*	*2.5*

Mean weight of bran contained in one heaping teaspoon
(largest heap possible) of those tested: 2.3

TABLESPOON REGULAR BRAN
HEAPING (SMALL HEAP)

(All weights in grams)	Stainless Steel	Round Plastic	Oval Plastic	Round Aluminum
Weight of container	10.2	10.2	10.2	10.2
Weight of container plus 10 heaping tbsp. bran (small heap)	61.4	56.8	66.7	70.9
Weight of 10 tbsp. bran alone	51.2	56.8	56.5	60.7
Weight of one heaping tbsp. bran (small heap)	5.1	4.7	5.7	6.1

Mean weight of bran contained in one heaping tablespoon
(small heap) of those tested: 5.4

TABLESPOON REGULAR BRAN
HEAPING (LARGEST HEAP POSSIBLE)

(All weights in grams)	Stainless Steel	Round Plastic	Oval Plastic	Round Aluminum
Weight of container	10.2	10.2	10.2	10.2
Weight of container plus 10 heaping tbsp. bran (largest heap possible)	85.0	73.2	66.7	70.9
Weight of 10 tbsp. bran alone	74.8	63.0	72.8	81.2
Weight of one heaping tbsp. bran (largest heap possible)	7.5	6.3	7.3	8.1

Mean weight of bran contained in one heaping tablespoon
(largest heap possible) of those tested: 7.3

TEASPOON FINE BRAN
HEAPING (SMALL HEAP)

(All weights in grams)	Stainless Steel	Round Plastic	Oval Plastic	Round Aluminum
Weight of container	10.2	10.2	10.2	10.2
Weight of container plus 10 heaping tsp. fine bran (small heap)	36.9	32.7	36.4	35.8
Weight of 10 tsp. fine bran alone	26.7	22.5	26.2	25.6
Weight of one heaping tsp. fine bran (small heap)	2.7	2.3	2.6	2.6

Mean weight of fine bran contained in one heaping teaspoon (small heap) of those tested: 2.6

TEASPOON FINE BRAN
HEAPING (LARGEST HEAP POSSIBLE)

(All weights in grams)	Stainless Steel	Round Plastic	Oval Plastic	Round Aluminum
Weight of container	10.2	10.2	10.2	10.2
Weight of container plus 10 heaping tsp. fine bran (largest heap possible)	64.2	47.7	56.9	53.3
Weight of 10 tsp. fine bran alone	54.0	37.5	46.7	43.1
Weight of one heaping tsp. fine bran (largest heap possible)	5.4	3.8	4.7	4.3

Mean weight of fine bran contained in one heaping teaspoon (largest heap possible) of those tested: 4.6

TABLESPOON FINE BRAN
HEAPING (SMALL HEAP)

(All weights in grams)	Stainless Steel	Round Plastic	Oval Plastic	Round Aluminum
Weight of container	*10.2*	*10.2*	*10.2*	*10.2*
Weight of container plus 10 heaping tbsp. fine bran (small heap)	*70.9*	*69.6*	*72.2*	*78.2*
Weight of 10 tbsp. fine bran alone	*60.7*	*59.4*	*62.0*	*68.0*
Weight of one heaping tbsp. fine bran (small heap)	*6.1*	*5.9*	*6.2*	*6.8*

Mean weight of fine bran contained in one heaping tablespoon (small heap) of those tested: 6.3

TABLESPOON FINE BRAN
HEAPING (LARGEST HEAP POSSIBLE)

(All weights in grams)	Stainless Steel	Round Plastic	Oval Plastic	Round Aluminum
Weight of container	*10.2*	*10.2*	*10.2*	*10.2*
Weight of container plus 10 heaping tbsp. fine bran (largest heap possible)	*107.4*	*98.9*	*106.7*	*121.8*
Weight of 10 tbsp. fine bran alone	*97.2*	*88.7*	*96.5*	*111.6*
Weight of one heaping tbsp. fine bran (largest heap possible)	*9.7*	*8.9*	*9.7*	*11.2*

Mean weight of fine bran contained in one heaping tablespoon (largest heap possible) of those tested: 9.9

How to Make Fine Bran

In my area of the country unprocessed bran can only be found in health-food stores. It is not to be confused with the sugar-containing bran cereals that are sold under various trade names in the supermarket. You may find unprocessed bran labeled as Crude Bran, Pure Bran, Coarse Bran, Miller's Bran, or Bran Flakes. In general, the various brands in health-food stores seem to be identical. It is a very inexpensive substance.

Throughout the book and in the recipes I make reference to fine bran. This will have to be made by the reader by grinding regular bran in a small, inexpensive electric food mill. The stores in my area sell four different types. They range in price from about $12 to about $20. Some are sold as coffee-bean grinders, but work quite well for the purpose suggested here. They are very quick and simple to use. The four that I am aware of are

- the Salton Food Mill
- the Braun Coffee Mill
- the Moulinex Coffee Mill
- the Bialetti Rollmix

Keep in mind that fine bran, because it is more concentrated, is used in a ratio of two heaping tablespoons for each three heaping tablespoons of regular bran.

APPENDIX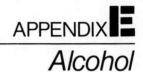

Alcohol

Alcohol contains nothing but naked calories. There is not a bit of fiber in it, nor can any be added. On the reducing diet it is forbidden at all times.

It is presumptuous for me to tell you that you can't have it, ever, on The Weight-Maintenance Diet, but that is what I would like to tell you. If you must have a drink on The Weight-Maintenance Diet, then do your weight a big favor and have no more than one drink a day. It can be either before, during, or after dinner. But whatever you do, do not use sweet mixers, which are in essence soft drinks with sugar in them.

NOTES ON SCIENTIFIC BACKGROUND AND SOURCES

CHAPTER TWO

Dr. Cleave's statement that no birth defect is present in more than 0.5 percent of the population appeared in T. L. Cleave, *The Saccharine Disease* (Bristol, 1974, p. 2). Additional reference on this point is made in F. Grundy and E. Lewis-Fanning, *Morbidity and Mortality in the First Year of Life* (London, Eugenics Society). Estimates of the exact incidence of obesity in the Western world vary because statistics on this point are not commonly collected. One estimate can be found in Beeson and McDermott, *Textbook of Medicine* (Saunders, 1975, p. 1375).

The absence of obesity among Zulu tribes living in rural Natal, South Africa is reviewed in C. Slome, B. Gampel, J. H. Abrahamson, and N. Scotch, *South African Medical Journal,* Vol. 34 (1960), p. 505, as well as Cleave (1974, p. 76). The dietary evaluation of the Zulus is discussed by a number of researchers. Their consumption of 90 percent carbohydrates is pointed out by A. M. Lubbe, "Dietary Evaluation," *South African Medical Journal,* Vol. 45 (1971), pp. 1289–1297. Their consumption of sugarcane is in G. D. Campbell, *South African Medical Journal,* Vol. 37 (1963), p. 1195. Further dietary evaluation is found in T. L. Cleave, G. D. Campbell, and N. S. Painter, *Diabetes, Coronary Thrombosis and the Saccharine Disease,* 2nd edition (Bristol, 1969), and J. H. Cummings, "Progress Report, Dietary Fibre," *Gut,* Vol. 14 (1973), pp. 68–81. The incidence of obesity in Zulu men and women living in urban areas is presented in C. Slome and others, *South African Medical Journal,* Vol. 34, p. 506. Comparisons of the diet of urban Zulus with rural Zulus are offered in G. D. Campbell, *South African Medical Journal,* Vol. 34 (1960), p. 332; in Cleave (1974, pp. 86–87); and in G. D. Campbell, *South African Medical Journal,* Vol. 37 (1963), p. 1199. The comparative consumption of over 100 pounds of sugar per year by Americans is found in Berta Friend, "Nutrients in U. S. Food Supply," *American Journal of Clinical Nutrition,* Vol. 20 (1967), pp. 907–914, and U. S. Food Consumption, Sources of Data and Trends, pp. 1909–1963, *Statistical Bulletin #364 and Supplement* (Washington, D. C.: U. S. Department of Agriculture, 1965). The health differences between urban and rural Zulus is presented in A. Barker, *Lancet,* Vol. 2 (1964), p. 970, and in H. C. Seftel and K. J. Keeley, *South African Medical Journal,* Vol. 37 (1963), p. 1213.

The switch from brown sugar to white sugar in the latter half of the nineteenth century in the U. S. is reviewed in Richard O. Cummings, *The American and His Food,* chapter 8, "An Indefinable Loss" (New York, 1970); in John Searles, "American Sugar," in *One Hundred Years of American Commerce,* Chauncey Depew, ed. (New York, 1895, pp. 258–260); and in George Sorface, *The Story of Sugar* (New York, 1910, pp. 178 ff). The monopolization of the sugar industry by 1900 is given in Cummings (1970, pp. 111–112), and House Hearings before The Special Committee on the Investigation of the American Sugar Refining Co. (62nd Congress, 2nd Session, July 17, 1911, pp. 1864–1865). The history of the increase in Great Britain's per capita sugar consumption are compiled from M. A. Antar, et al., *American Journal of Clinical Nutrition,* Vol. 14 (1964), pp. 169–178, and the *Journal of the Royal Naval Medical Service,* Vol. 42 (1956), #2, p. 55, and Cleave (1974, p. 7). The doubling of sugar consumption in the United States, and its rise to 120 pounds per person per year are in M. A. Antar, et al., *American Journal of Clinical Nutrition,* Vol. 14 (1964), pp. 169–178.

The change in the technology for milling wheat at the end of the nineteenth century appears in Charles Kuhlman, *The Development of the Flour Milling Industry in the U. S.* (Boston, 1929, pp. 114, 120–123), and Cummings (1970, p. 113). The decline in the use of flour in America at the turn of the century is reviewed by the *U. S. Dept. of Agriculture Yearbook* (1921, p. 159), and by Cummings (1970, Appendix B). The enrichment of white bread with vitamins required by government because of refining is discussed by Marie V. Krause, *Food Nutrition and Diet Therapy* (Philadelphia, 1972, p. 52).

The 25-gram per day fiber intake of rural Zulus is in a variety of research reports. Two of the recent ones are A. M. Lubbe, *South African Medical Journal,* Vol. 45 (1971), pp. 1289–1297, and J. H. Cummings, *Gut,* Vol. 14 (1973), pp. 69–81. The 3- to 5-gram quantity of fiber eaten by Americans is discussed in Cummings (1973), and in M. G. Hardinge, et al., "Dietary Levels of Fiber," *American Journal of Clinical Nutrition,* Vol. 6, pp. 523–525. The interested reader might want to study J. Robertson, "Changes in the Fibre Content of the British Diet," *Nature* (London), Vol. 238 (1972), pp. 290–292.

CHAPTER THREE

The twenty-four- to forty-eight-hour transit time of rural Zulus is reported on by O. N. Mandusos, S. C. Truelove, and K. Lumsden, *British Medical Journal,* Vol. 3 (1967), p. 760; by D. P. Burkitt, A. R. P. Walker, and J. S. Painter, *Lancet,* Vol. 2 (1972), p. 1408; and by Cleave (1974, p. 28). Studies that report that the transit time in the Western world is forty-eight to ninety-six hours include the same three sources. The study that analyzed 1,000 subjects from varying ethnic backgrounds and showed that the more refined the diet the smaller the stool and the longer the transit time is presented in the Burkitt, et al., reference cited above.

The 10-percent prevalence of varicose veins in the American population is discussed in R. R. Foote, *Varicose Veins,* 2nd edition (London, 1952, p. 38); in Cleave (1974, pp. 44–45); and in D. P. Burkett, *British Medical Journal,* Vol. 2 (1972), pp. 556–561.

An explanation of the mechanism by which the hard stool of the refined diet causes varicose veins is in Cleave (1974, p. 48). The hospital in the Zululand Reserve that had only 3 reported cases of varicose veins out of over 100,000 admissions for three years is in H. Dodd, *Lancet,* Vol. 2 (1964), p. 809. The equivalent incidence of varicose veins between the white and black populations of the U. S. is presented in J. H. Lewis *The Biology of the Negro* (Chicago, 1942), and in T. L. Cleave and G. D. Campbell (1966, 1st edition). The hospital that had 30,000 patients but only 1 case of varicosities is reported by D. P. Burkitt (1972, pp. 556–561). This article also included his personal examination of 4,000 adults in central Africa, among whom he found only 5 cases of varicose veins. The medical questionnaire sent to 114 hospitals in Africa is reported in the same article, as is the review of hospitals in India and Pakistan. The study of 9,000 patients in Iran which showed a complete absence of leg ulcer is in W. A. D. Griffiths, *British Medical Journal,* Vol. 2 (1972), p. 770. The post-operative care of patients with a high-fiber diet is reported by both Cleave (1974, p. 127–128) and by C. Latto, *British Medical Journal,* Vol. 3 (1972), p. 705.

Studies that indicate that diverticular disease affects one person out of every three over age forty-five, and two out of three over age eighty include T. G. Parks, *Proceedings of the Royal Society of Medicine,* Vol. 61 (1968), p. 932, and L. E. Hughes, *Gut,* Vol. 10 (1969), pp. 336–351. The thirty- to forty-year incubation period for diverticulosis is presented in Cleave (1974, p. 33) and in N. S. Painter and D. P. Burkitt, *British Medical Journal,* Vol. 2 (1971), p. 450. The latter article includes Dr. Burkitt's statement that in twenty years of surgery in African hospitals he never saw a case of diverticulosis (p. 452). Also discussed was the dramatic increase of diverticular disease during the last seventy years. The hospital in Kampala, Africa, that reported only 2 cases in 4,000 autopsies is in H. C. Trowell, *Non-Infective Diseases in Africa* (London, 1960).

The fact that heart disease is the greatest single cause of

illness and premature death in most Western nations is pointed out in T. W. Meade and R. Chakrabarti, *Lancet,* Vol. 2 (1972), p. 913, and by Beeson and McDermott (1975, p. 992). The latter reference also reports that heart disease takes more lives than respiratory illnesses, cerebral vascular disease, and accidents. U. Schire, in the *South African Medical Journal,* Vol. 45, pp. 634–644, states that the most common kind of heart attack is the result of coronary artery disease. The crude death rate that shows that heart disease takes twice as many lives as cancer is reported in the *Statistical Abstract of the United States* (Washington, U. S. Dept. of Commerce, 1972, pp. 59–60). Historical review of the increase in the per capita consumption of vegetable fat in this country is discussed in B. Friend (1967, p. 907), in Cleave (1974, p. 20), and in Antar, et al. (1964, p. 169). Both Cleave and Antar, et al., point out the small amount of change in the amount of animal fats eaten by individuals in this country. The rapid rise in the death rate from coronary disease in this country over the last fifty to sixty years is covered by C. K. Friedberg, *Disease of the Heart,* 3rd edition (Philadelphia, 1966, p. 771); by H. Trowell, N. S. Painter, and D. Burkitt, *Digestive Disease,* Vol. 19 (1974), p. 864; and in the September 6, 1974, article, "Roughage in the Diet" in *Medical World News,* pp. 35–42. The worldwide parallel between the incidence of coronary artery disease and diverticular disease is reported in both Cleave (1974, p. 107), and by T. W. Meade and R. Chakrabarti (1972, p. 913). The forty-year incubation period for coronary artery disease is discussed in Cleave (1974, p. 107). As to specific examples, the high consumption of animal fats by Eskimos is reported in O. Schaefer, *Nutrition Today,* Vol. 6 (1971), No. 6, p. 8, and in Cleave (1974, p. 113). The eleven-year study at the Baragwanath Hospital that showed only 30 admissions for coronary artery disease is reported in H. C. Seftel, et al. (1963, p. 148). The Bantu Hospital in Pretoria that reported only nine cases of coronary artery disease in three years, the reports from 137 hospitals in 20 African countries, and the 94 African doctors that stated they had never diagnosed a case of coronary artery disease are all presented in H. Trowell, N. S. Painter, and D. Burkitt, *Digestive Disease,* Vol. 19 (1974), p. 864. This article also points out the large incidence of coronary artery disease in Africa's large cities where the diet is Westernized, as do U. Schrire (1971, pp. 634–644), and H. C. Seftel, M. C. Kew, and I. Bersohn, *South African Medical Journal,* Vol. 44 (1970), pp. 8–12. The report on Dr. Burkitt's questionnaire, sent to 36 hospitals in high-fiber eating areas of India and Pakistan, is found in S. L. M. Malhotra, *British Heart Journal,* Vol. 29 (1967), p. 337. This is also the 1967 *British Medical Journal* article that reported that a group of railway workers in southern India ate little animal fat but had a high incidence of coronary artery disease. *The British Medical Journal* article that reported that coronary artery disease is seldom seen in Africans who were obese, had hypertension, or had diabetes is by A. G. Shaper, and appears in Vol. 4, p. 32. The study that compared the Irish men with their brothers in Boston is in H. Trowell, *Proceedings of the Nutrition Society,* Vol. 32 (1973), p. 151. Dr. John Yudkin's epidemiological evidence as to the correlation of sugar consumption and coronary disease is from his book, *Sweet and Dangerous* (New York, pp. 94–101).

A topic of particular interest to many readers is the relationship between fiber and the diet and cholesterol levels in the blood. My statement in the book that a high-fiber diet lowers blood cholesterol has a number of studies which support it, and among them are the following: M. A. Eastwood, et al., "The Effects of Dietary Supplement of Wheat Bran and Cellulose on Faeces," *Proceedings of the Nutrition Society,* Vol. 32 (1973), p. 22A; K. S. Shurpacekar, et al., "Effect of inclusion of cellulose in an 'Atherogenic' Diet on the Blood Lipids of Children," *Nature* (London), Vol. 232 (1971), pp. 554–555; A. . de Groot et al., "Cholesterol-Lowering Effect of Rolled Oats," *Cancer,* Vol. 2 (1963), pp. 303–304; K. S. Hathur et al., "Hypocholesterol effect of Bengal Gram: A Long-term Study in Man," *British Medical Journal,* Vol. 1 (1968), pp. 30–31; C. H. Edwards, et al., "Utilization of Wheat by Adult Man: Nitrogen Metabolism,

Plasma Amino Acids, and Lipids," *American Journal of Clinical Nutrition,* Vol. 24 (1971), pp. 181–193; R. Loyken et al., "The Influences of Legumes on the Serum Cholesterol Level," *Uoeding,* Vol. 23 (1962), pp. 447–453; A. Keys, et al., "Diet Type (Fats Constant) and Blood Lipids in Man," *Journal of Nutrition,* Vol. 70 (1960), pp. 257–266; A. Keys, "Fiber and Pectin in the Diet and Serum Cholesterol Concentration in Man," *Proceedings of the Society for Experimental Biology and Medicine,* Vol. 106 (1961), pp. 555–558; J. J. Groen, "Why Bread in the Diet Lowers Serum Cholesterol," *Proceedings of the Nutrition Society,* Vol. 32 (1973), pp. 159–167.

Historical data on peptic ulcer is available in Dr. Cleave's book, *Peptic Ulcer* (Wright, 1962). The percentage of Britons who have clinically diagnosed ulcers, and the percentages found in autopsies after death, are given in W. R. S. Doll, F. A. Jones, and M. M. Buckatzsch, *Spec. Rep. Serv. Med. Research Council* (1950), London, No. 276, and by Cleave (1974, p. 139). The statistic on the Charles Johnson Memorial Hospital in Nqutu where only two cases of peptic ulcer were observed in ten years is a personal communication form A. Barker to Cleave (1974, p. 150). The government radiologist in Ethiopia who reported an incidence of peptic ulcer of two per thousand is a personal communication to Cleave (1962, p. 31) as is the high incidence of peptic ulcer in Addis Ababa. The statistic of only two cases of peptic ulcer at Wusasa Hospital in Nigeria is reported by Cleave (1974, p. 151). The U. S. Army report that peptic ulcer has become as common in blacks as in whites is in A. A. Kirschner, *Review of Gastroenterology,* Vol. 11 (1944), p. 397, which contrasts with the less common incidence of this in blacks fifty or so years ago as compared to whites, previously reported in U. Maes and E. McFetridge, *American Journal of Surgery,* Vol. 33 (1936), p. 5. The buffering action of protein on hydrochloric acid is covered by Cleave in both of his books (1974, pp. 140–144) and (1962, p. 134). The removal of protein by refining from unprocessed foods, particularly wheat, rice, and the peeling and boiling of potatoes is in R. A. McCance and E. M. Widdowson, *The Chemical Composition of Foods,* 3rd edition (London, 1960). X-ray studies showing that eating different foods one at a time produces a layering effect of foods in the stomach is reported by both N. A. Nielson and H. Christiansen, *Acta Radiologica,* Vol. 13 (1932), p. 678, and Cleave (1974, p. 143). The 1968 article in *Gut* that showed that stomach acidity increased more after eating refined grain than eating unrefined grain is by Lennard-Jones, Fletcher, and Shaw, and is in Vol. 9, p. 177. Data about prisoner-of-war camps in the Far East is in J. Taylor, *History of Second World War,* U. K. Medical Series, The Royal Naval Medical Service; Surgery, Sir Zachary Cope, editor (London, p. 744). Additional evidence on war prisoners in the Far East can be found in H. L. Cleave, *Journal of the Royal Naval Medical Service,* Vol. 44 (1958), p. 77. Data about German soldiers who served on the Russian front is from Cleave (1962, p. 64). The other reports that cover the situation of the German soldiers on the Russian front include H. Glatzel, *Ergebn. Inn Med. Kinderheilk,* Vol. 65 (1945), p. 504, and H. Glatzel, *Aretl. Wschr.,* Vol. 2 (1952), p. 1063.

One book which describes the location of tooth decay below the gum line in ancient peoples is by W. A. Price, *Nutrition and Physical Degeneration* (Los Angeles, American Academy of Applied Nutrition, 1950). The sudden increase in tooth decay in 1932 on the island of Tristan da Cunha is reported by F. B. Gamblan, *Journal of the Royal Naval Medical Service,* Vol. 39 (1953), No. 4, p. 252.

Dr. John Yudkin's position on the relationship between eating too much sugar and the incidence of diabetes can be found in his book, *Sweet and Dangerous,* pp. 113–121. The consumption of over four ounces of refined sugar a day by the average American can be found in M. A. Antar, et al. (1964, pp. 169–178). A discussion of the Natal Indians in South Africa who eat over 110 pounds of sugar per person per year, contrasting their high rate of diabetes with the low rate of rural Zulus who live in the same area and eat very little refined carbohydrate, is reported in S. L. M. Malhotra, *British Heart Journal,* Vol. 29 (1967), p. 337, and in G. D. Campbell (1963, p. 1195). The former article, by Malhotra, also reports on southern India, where the diet is milled white rice and the incidence of diabetes is high. The latter article, by Campbell, points out that urine tests on 2,000 sugarcane cutters in Africa showed sugar in only three. The report by Dr. Frederick Banting that of 5,000 native workers on the Panama Canal, only two had sugar in their urine while native Spaniards in the same area, who ate refined sugar, had a high incidence of diabetes, is discussed by Banting himself in the *Edinburgh Medical Journal,* Vol. 36, January (1929), p. 1. Dr. A. M. Cohen's study of Jews who emigrated to Israel from three widely separated parts of the world, and their diabetic histories, is reported in A. M. Cohen, S. Bauly, and R. Poznanski, *Lancet,* Vol. 2 (1961), p. 1399. The rising incidence of diabetes among Canadian Eskimos who recently started eating more sugar is presented in O. Shaefer (1971, p. 8). The absence of diabetes among the Greenland Eskimos who do not eat sugar is covered in H. O. Barg, J. Dyerberg, and A. B. Nielsen, *Lancet* (1971), p. 1143. The lower incidence of diabetes among blacks than among East Indians in Trinidad is reported in T. Poon-King, M. V. Henry, and F. Rampersad, *Lancet* (1968), Vol. 1, p. 155. The change in the eating of sugar and the rising incidence of diabetes in Iceland is covered in V. Albertsson, *Diabetes* (1953), Vol. 2, p. 184.

Dr. Denis Burkitt's statement that a number of diseases have a common cause, which is the absence of fiber, is presented in "The Evidence Leavens: We Invite Colon Cancer," *Medical World News,* August 11, 1972, p. 33. The recovery abilities of the body as expressed in the smoking versus lung cancer situation are shown by those who quit nearly eliminating the chance of contracting lung cancer are stated in the *U. S. Surgeon General's Advisory Committee on Smoking and Health* (1964), p. 31. Studies on smokers that show that within six to nine months after quitting the appearance of the lungs improves are reported in G. James and T. Rosenthal, editors, *Tobacco and*

Health (Springfield, 1962, p. 97), and in H. S. Diehl, *Tobacco and Your Health: The Smoking Controversy* (New York, 1969, pp. 135–136). The current fact that one third of those who contract cancer today survive is covered in the National Cancer Institute, Third National Cancer Survey. A discussion of polyps of the colon will be found in Harrison's *Principles of Internal Medicine,* 7th edition (1974), p. 1492. Dr. Benjamin Ershoff's study on mice which established that fiber in their diet protects them from chemical substance in their food is very recent. It can be found in B. H. Ershoff, *American Journal of Clinical Nutrition,* Vol. 27 (1974), p. 1395.

CHAPTER FIVE

The British experiment that showed that it takes longer to eat whole wheat bread than white bread is reported in R. A. McCance et al. (1953, p. 98), in D. P. Burkitt, *Proceedings of the Nutrition Society,* Vol. 32 (1973), p. 145, and in Cleave (1974, p. 148). Reports that the average American consumes 3 to 5 grams daily include M. G. Hardinge, et al. (1958, pp. 523–525), and J. H. Cummings (1973, pp. 69–81).

INDEX